PREGNANCY
& PARENTHOOD

The National Childbirth Trust is a registered charity which exists to further education for parenthood. The views expressed in this book are those of the authors and do not necessarily reflect those of the Trust or the publishers.

Pregnancy & Parenthood has been compiled and prepared by Anne Loader, in cooperation with Eileen Hutton, Deirdre Y. Mackay, and Margaret B. Duncan Shearer.

List of contributors:

Janet Backhouse
Bridget Baker
Josephine Burns
Margaret Ellison
Rosemary Fost
Professor Peter Huntingford
Sheila Kitzinger
Belinda Lee-Jones

Dr. Michael Lee-Jones
Anne Loader
Geraldine Lux Flanagan
Dr. James Aidan MacFarlane
Deirdre Y. Mackay
Christina Paulson-Ellis
Dr. N. R. C. Roberton
Gwen Rankin
Margaret Williams

In addition members of the following three National Childbirth Trust Committees have helped in the compilation of this book: The Breastfeeding Promotion Group, the Technical Committee, and the Teacher's Panel. Elizabeth Cook compiled the Index.

Drawings by Nigel Casseldine

ACKNOWLEDGEMENTS

Diagrams on pp. 79 (top), 80, 82, 83, 84 based on material in M. Williams and D. Booth, *Antenatal Education* (Churchill Livingstone, 1974). Acknowledgement is also made to Maternity Center Association, New York, whose *Birth Atlas* provided the basis for the drawings on pp. 11, 67, 70, 71, 73, 74, 75, 76; and to R. J. Demarest and J. J. Sciarra, *Conception, Birth and Contraception* (1969) which was also used for anatomical reference.

PREGNANCY
& PARENTHOOD

edited by Anne Loader
on behalf of the
National Childbirth Trust

Oxford · New York · Toronto · Melbourne
OXFORD UNIVERSITY PRESS
1980

Oxford University Press, Walton Street, Oxford OX2 6DP

Oxford   London   Glasgow
New York   Toronto   Melbourne   Wellington
Kuala Lumpur   Singapore   Jakarta   Hong Kong   Tokyo
Delhi   Bombay   Calcutta   Madras   Karachi
Nairobi   Dar es Salaam   Cape Town

British Library Cataloguing in Publication Data
National Childbirth Trust
Pregnancy and parenthood. – (Popular medical).
1. Pregnancy
2. Childbirth
I. Title   II. Series
612.6'3   RG524   79–41284

ISBN 0-19-217684-6
ISBN 0-19-286006-2 Pbk

Typeset by Filmtype Services Limited, Scarborough
Printed in Great Britain by Cox & Wyman Ltd, Reading

Foreword

The National Childbirth Trust has played a major role in the development of education for childbirth and parenthood in this country. For many years it has pioneered, and campaigned for, the wider provision of adequate preparation classes for labour. Even today a great deal of this important aspect of maternity care is still provided by the dedicated members of the NCT.

It is therefore very right and proper that they should produce a book which reflects the accumulated experience and knowledge of their many very accomplished childbirth educators, as well as some of their professional advisers. Parts of this book are based on several short publications which have been issued separately during the past few years.

No one can pretend there is a shortage of baby books currently available on the market. However, there can be few which bring such a comprehensive, practical, and realistic outline of the problems associated with pregnancy, labour, and the puerperium. This book will certainly be read with enormous interest by mothers from all over this country as well as overseas. It will form a most valuable contribution to the expanding programme of preventative obstetric care which must be concerned with the emotional just as much as with the physical problems of childbirth.

Norman Morris, MD, FRCOG,
Professor of Obstetrics and Gynaecology,
Charing Cross Hospital Medical School.

CONTENTS

PREGNANCY

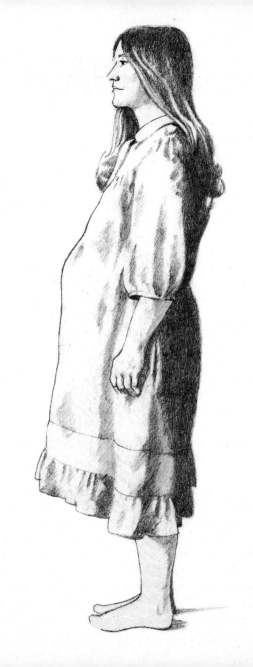

Introduction

Most women know little about pregnancy until they embark on it for the first time. If you have planned the pregnancy, you may well be more knowledgeable about contraception than about the conception and development of the foetus you are carrying. Some of the outward signs of early pregnancy, as they affect the mother, are well known – missed periods, morning sickness, and tiredness – but little emphasis is placed on the concurrent fascinating development of the unborn child, which is recognizably human from a very early stage and is remarkably complex. And however much you know in theory about pregnancy and parenthood, actually experiencing it is something new for each individual.

During the nine months of pregnancy the baby's bodily systems mature to the point where he can sustain life independent of the womb. Although at first you can be quite unaware of being pregnant, later you are constantly aware of the baby as he takes up more room in your body and his kicks and stretchings become stronger. Throughout pregnancy, the two of you are bound up together: the changes in his body directly cause changes in yours, and your health affects his development.

The culmination of pregnancy is giving birth. It is sensible for you to learn how to make this climax as rewarding as possible for yourself and as easy as possible for the baby. To do this you can learn relaxation and breathing patterns which will help your body to work more efficiently during labour, as well as distracting you from the power of your labour, or contractions.

In order to check that everything is going well with the pregnancy, you should take full advantage of the comprehensive antenatal care available to all expectant mothers in this country. You and your baby both benefit from these check-ups, inconvenient though they may sometimes be.

Pregnancy affects the physical and emotional aspects of sexuality. The key to most problems of this nature is patience, linked with a willingness to explore new ways of lovemaking, and an understanding of what causes these temporary difficulties.

However much you have longed for a baby, there are always adjustments to be made when a couple is in the process of being transformed into a family. It is often hard for a woman to accept what she may regard as the 'inferior' role of motherhood, after the stimulus and responsibility of a full-time job. But the more you learn about it, the more you will come to realize how challenging and stimulating parenthood can be. You will also be in a position to make the best possible decisions for yourself and your baby.

This book is written for fathers as well as mothers. At last it has become respectable for men to take an active caring interest in their wives' pregnancies (though they have probably done so throughout history, albeit less openly than they do now), and for them to provide invaluable help and support when their children are born.

Conception and development of the foetus

Your baby began as a single cell; when he is born, roughly 266 days later, this one cell will have multiplied to have become 200 million highly specialized cells in the complex body of a tiny human being.

In a sense, each new life has no definite beginning. Its existence is inherent in the existence of the parent cells and these, in turn, have arisen from the preceding parent cells. When any two parent cells unite, they bring together a blend of the attributes of all ancestors before them. Your baby is a completely new individual – not just a mixture of his parents' features but of characteristics which can be traced back through many generations. He is a link with the past and with the future.

The egg and the sperm

The female egg comes from the mother's ovary. She has two ovaries, each containing about a quarter of a million immature egg cells. Normally, one egg ripens each month in alternate ovaries, approximately two weeks before a menstrual period. The ripe egg bursts out of the ovary and falls into the trumpet-shaped opening of the Fallopian tube, which has an internal diameter the thickness of a cat's whisker and is about 10 cm (4 in) long. One tube leads from each ovary to the thimble-sized cavity of the uterus, or womb. The minute round egg is slowly wafted towards the uterus by a gentle current of fluids within the tube. The egg has a very brief life and disintegrates unless it is fertilized and activated by a male cell on the first or second day after its arrival in the tube.

The male cells, or sperm, are produced in the father's testicles. At least 20 million and often as many as 500 million sperm cells may be present in a single ejaculation, but probably only a few dozen of the original millions released during inter-course ever reach the egg, high up in the Fallopian tube. The male cells are much smaller than the egg and are often likened to miniature tadpoles because they look similar and can swim by lashing their tails backwards and forwards. It has been estimated that some male cells can travel the 17-cm (7-in) distance from the vagina to the Fallopian tubes in a little over an hour. A powerful enzyme helps one sperm to 'eat' its way through the outer membrane of the egg, then through a finer underlying membrane holding the substance of the egg, until it reaches the centre and fuses with the maternal cell nucleus. Then a coating forms round the fertilized egg and prevents other sperm cells from entering.

In the nuclei of the sperm and the egg there are many thousands of genes which carry the 'instructions' or specifica-tions for the design of every part of the new baby. With so many genes there can obviously be a virtually infinite number of variations on exisiting family patterns.

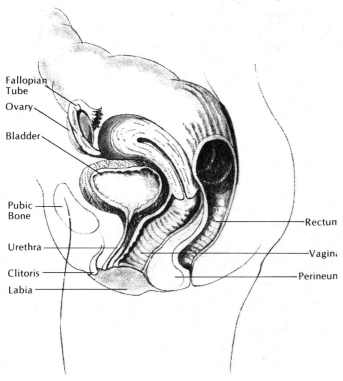

Fallopian
Tube
Ovary
Bladder
Pubic
Bone
Urethra
Clitoris
Labia

Rectum
Vagina
Perineum

The female reproductive organs

The first three months

By the end of the first week the original two cells which fused to
form the fertilized egg, have multiplied into a cluster of more
than a hundred cells and have become implanted in the inner
lining of the uterus. (If no egg is implanted in this lining, it disintegrates and is shed with the unfertilized egg during menstruation.)

By the end of the first month a complete, recognizable
embryo has formed. It is only one centimetre ($\frac{1}{4}-\frac{1}{2}$ in) long but
already has a head with rudimentary eyes, ears, mouth, and a

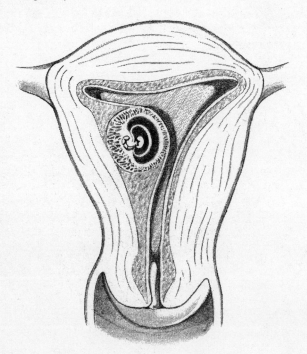

6-week embryo (actual size)

brain. It has simple kidneys, a liver, a digestive tract, a primitive umbilical cord, the beginnings of a beating heart, and its own bloodstream. It is surrounded by an amnion or bag of waters, and is enclosed in a capsule covered with hundreds of root-like tufts which channel food from the lining of the uterus.

By the seventh week the embryo bears the familiar features and all the internal organs of the future adult, even though he is only 2 cm (less than an inch) long and weighs about a gramme ($\frac{1}{30}$ oz). He has a human face with eyes, ears, nose, lips, tongue, and even milk teeth buds in the gums. The body has become rounded, padded with muscles, and covered by a thin skin. The tiny arms have hands with fingers and thumbs, and the slower-

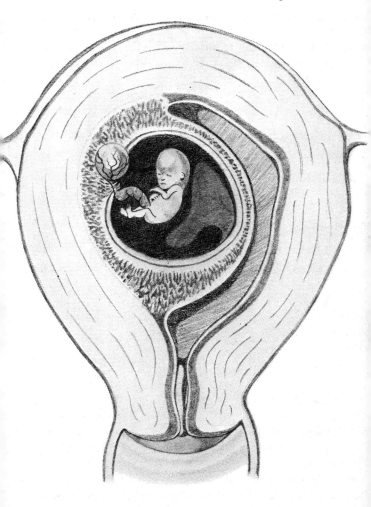

10-week embryo (actual size)

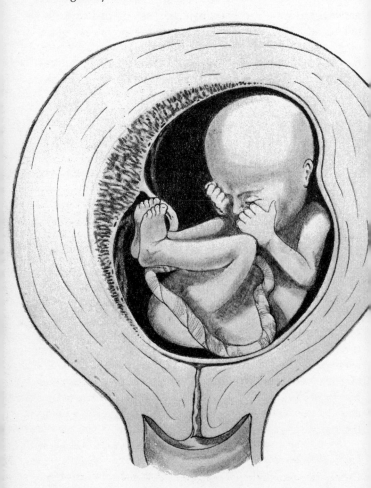

14-week baby in the uterus, showing placenta (actual size)

growing legs have recognizable knees, ankles, and toes. The brain sends out impulses to co-ordinate the functioning of the other organs and the muscles of the arms and body can already be set in motion. The heart beats sturdily, the stomach produces digestive juices, the liver manufactures blood cells, and the kidneys extract uric acid from the blood.

During this period of teeming cell growth, the new cells are especially vulnerable to all physical and chemical influences, and diseases can be communicated from the mother. For this reason you should avoid exposure to known infectious diseases, take no drugs without medical advice, and avoid X-rays. It is wise to avoid these risks altogether as soon as you are planning to conceive, or think you have conceived, a child, even before you have missed a period. To some extent nature provides its own cure: if an embryo fails to grow properly, the 'mistake' is often rectified by an early miscarriage.

During the third month after conception, the baby begins to be quite active, although he is still so tiny that he would easily fit into a goose's egg and weighs only 28 g (1 oz). You are very unlikely to be able to feel your baby's movements because he is so small that the uterus has barely expanded and is still contained within the girdle of your hip-bones. However, by the end of the third month he can kick his legs, turn his feet, curl and fan his toes, make a fist, move his thumb, open his mouth, and press his lips tightly together. He will swallow considerable amounts of amniotic fluid and may even 'breathe' it in and out of his primitive lungs.

From the fourth to the six month

During the fourth to fifth month you will probably feel the baby turning and kicking against your sensitive abdominal wall. The uterus will have risen out of the confines of your pelvis and the baby will be much stronger. These first-perceived movements are called 'quickening' and can be a very exciting milestone in your pregnancy. In the fourth month the baby grows so much that he reaches half the height he will be at birth. He becomes

20–25 cm (8–10 in) tall but still weighs only about 170 g (6 oz). He is nourished through the umbilical cord which is attached to the placenta, which in turn is rooted in the lining of the uterus. The placenta is the organ through which the immature foetus receives oxygen and nutrients from your body, and also immunizing antibodies to combat infection, some of them produced by the placenta itself. The placenta is the main source of the hormones produced by your body in pregnancy which prepare for birth and the production of milk. Substances like alcohol, nicotine, and other drugs which enter your bloodstream may be transferred by the placenta to the baby within an hour or two.

In the fifth month the baby gains about 5 cm (2 in) in height and 28 g (10 oz) in weight. By the end of the month he will be about 30 cm (12 in) tall and will weigh about 500 g. Fine downy hair starts to grow, the skeleton hardens, and the nails begin to form. His heartbeat may be heard if an ear is placed next to your abdominal wall: fathers and siblings can now also feel him kicking, turning, and jerking rhythmically with hiccups. The baby will now find a characteristic position in which he prefers to sleep, but he may be stirred into activity by loud external noises or vibrations.

In the sixth month he will become about 35 cm (14 in) tall and will start to accumulate fat under his skin. His weight will increase to about 800 g (1¾ lb). He can open and close his eyes and develops a strong grip with his hands. He has a slim chance of surviving in an incubator if born prematurely.

The last three months

In these months the baby gains most of his birthweight and outgrows his home in the uterus. He usually puts on about 500 g (1 lb) in the seventh month and nearly 2 kg (4 lb) in the following six weeks. He develops a protective padding of fat which will help to keep his body warm after birth. He may begin to practise sucking (some babies are born with a callus on the thumb from sucking it *in utero*). He will probably settle into a head-down

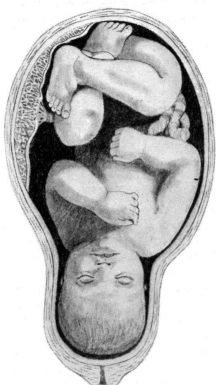

Fully-grown baby

position and his body will fill the uterus. When he moves the contours of his arms and legs can be felt and seen as bulges on your abdomen. During the last three months important immunizing agents to the diseases you have had or have been immunized against are transferred from you to the baby in the form of antibodies. These may be reinforced after birth by similar antibodies in your milk and its forerunner, colostrum. By the time these immunities wear off, at about six months of age, the baby's own system can cope better with infections and can begin to build up immunities of its own.

In the last month before birth, the expanded uterus sinks about 5 cm (2 in) downwards in your body and the baby's head (or buttocks) become engaged in the circle of your pelvic bones. This is called 'lightening' and will help to relieve the pressure of the baby underneath your rib-cage.

The baby's growth slows down as birth approaches – beautifully timed so that the baby becomes mature enough to be born just when he is still small enough to negotiate his exit.

Relaxation and muscle control in pregnancy and labour

As your figure changes and your baby grows, extra strain is put on some of your joints and muscles. This is due partly to the extra weight they must support and partly to a natural softening by the hormones which prepare your body for birth. A few simple excercises will help the muscles to become more supple but prevent them from becoming overstretched. Extra attention to the way you stand, sit, and move will prevent unnecessary strain, particularly on the joints of your back. During labour you will be able to control your muscles and breathing so that you can keep the rest of your body in harmony with the activities of your uterus.

Muscles and joints are not the only parts of your body that work harder during pregnancy; most of your internal organs are also more active. For example, your heart has to pump more blood round your body and your kidneys have to dispose of more waste matter. Most women are able to take these extra activities in their stride, but feel and look better if they live at a slightly slower pace and watch their diets with care.

With the approval of your doctor or midwife, exercises can be started after you are 16 weeks pregnant. It should only be necessary to spend about 10–15 minutes each day on the exercises, as several of the movements should become part of your daily lifestyle. Practise each exercise six times, counting four slowly as you do each movement and four as you return to your starting position. Provided there is no discomfort, always contract and relax each group of muscles as much as you can each time. *If you have any pain, bleeding, or minor illness, stop practising all the exercises until you have been medically examined.*

To prevent overstretching of the abdominal wall

Lie on your back with your knees bent and feet flat. Tighten your abdominal muscles so that the baby is pulled gently down towards your backbone. Relax slowly. Try to make a habit of tightening and relaxing your abdominal muscles in this way at intervals during the day when you are standing and sitting, particularly if you notice a 'sagging' feeling. If practised regularly this exercise is a great help towards getting your figure back after your baby is born.

To teach awareness (control) of the pelvic floor

A woman normally uses pelvic floor muscles around and deep inside the vagina during intercourse – often without being really aware of what she is doing. Increasing awareness of the actions of these muscles not only encourages relaxation during delivery and a quick recovery of muscle tone afterwards, but may also be helpful in your marriage. The following exercise will help you to locate and feel the muscles moving. Get into the same position as for the previous exercise, or sit on a low chair, leaning forward with your arms resting on your knees. Tighten the ring of muscles around your anus (back passage) as though you were trying to stop yourself passing a motion; make sure that your abdominal and buttock muscles remain relaxed. Let go. Now, tense then relax the muscles which surround the urethra and vagina (front passage and birth canal). You will be familiar with this sensation since it is the same as an internal kiss when you are making love. You use the same muscles when you need to pass water and are trying to hold on. A good test of their strength therefore is to try to 'stop the stream' for a moment when urinating. Now contract both sets of muscles together, thus pulling up the whole of the pelvic floor (the sling of muscle which surrounds the passages and supports your pelvic organs). Relax slowly and completely. Make this exercise another of your regular habits, particularly if you have to stand for some time and notice a heaviness between your legs.

Preparing for the birth of your baby's head

(a) Rest on your bed with your knees bent, your feet and knees wide apart, and your back supported by several pillows. Gradually relax your thighs and pelvic floor muscles so that your knees fall more and more widely apart (your feet will roll gently on to their outer borders). Leave your legs in this position. At first it may seem unnatural and uncomfortable, but after

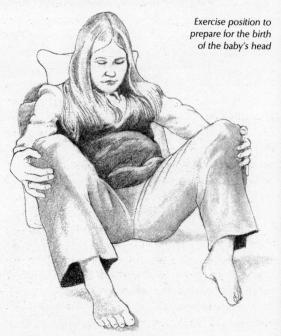

Exercise position to prepare for the birth of the baby's head

a little practice you will get the correct feeling of 'letting go' and can practise panting in this position, as you will be asked to do when it is time for your baby's head to pass slowly and gently out of the birth canal (see 'Breathing patterns', p. 77).

(b) Position yourself as for (a) but with your feet and knees together. Press your knees together hard and, at the same time, tighten the pelvic floor muscles as in the first exercise. Note the feeling of tension along the inner sides of your thighs and between your legs; many women do this involuntarily when their babies' heads are stretching the outlet of the birth canal. Relax, and notice carefully the different feel of the muscles; this is the feeling to aim for when you are giving birth.

To relieve backache

Sit on the front of a firm chair, leaning on your hands at the back of the seat. Hollow your back slightly; notice how your pelvis

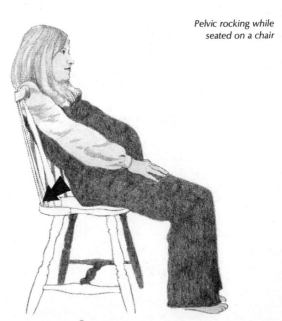

Pelvic rocking while seated on a chair

tilts down in front. Now round your back as much as you can; notice how your pelvis tilts up in front and your 'tail' is pulled well down at the back. Try the exercise standing up and lying down.

If you have backache, particularly the kind where you get 'locked' if you sit or lie for a long time, try 'unlocking' yourself by doing this pelvic rocking movement a few times before you attempt to change your position. If you suffer from backache during labour, try lying on your side and do the rocking very, very gently, in time with your breathing.

Active relaxation or decontraction

Lie on the floor with two or three cushions supporting your head and shoulders, a cushion in the small of your back, and your knees supported by a bolster or pillow. (Instead of these, a

Position for practising active decontraction, showing NCT 'wedge'

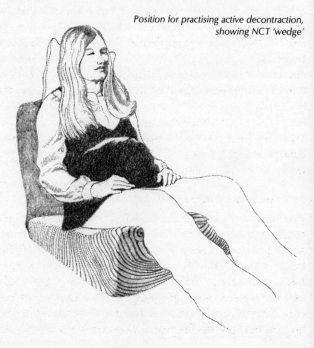

special 'wedge' is available from the NCT.) Tense all the muscles in your right arm and lift it a little way off the floor. Release the tension – that is, relax or 'decontract' the muscles – and the arm will fall to the ground like the arm of a puppet when the string is cut. Try again, but this time tense the muscles as if you were going to lift the arm but do not actually move it. Release the tension, noticing the different sensations. Repeat this tension and release with the muscles of the left arm, each leg, back, abdomen, pelvic floor, and face. Notice that when you tense you tend to hold your breath and when you relax you tend to breathe out. Finally, breathe in, hold your breath and make your whole body tense; breathe out and release every bit of tension in all the muscles of your body. Ask your husband to pick up an arm or leg and make sure that it remains heavy and relaxed even when it is moved. It is useful to practise these alternate contractions and decontractions so that you teach your brain to appreciate the different sensations coming from your muscles, but when you are actually in labour and your uterus begins to contract you will have time only to breathe in, breathe out, and let go all tension in the rest of your body immediately. Practise this speedy, complete relaxation in different positions; lying on your side, sitting in a chair leaning back or leaning forward with your head resting on a pile of pillows on a table. Try to use your new skill in everyday life. When coping with a difficult situation, meet it by breathing out and relaxing; you will find it much easier to deal with.

Selective relaxation or disassociation

When you find general relaxation easy you are ready to go one stage further. In labour it will be much harder to tolerate a strong contraction of your uterus and still relax the rest of your body, because muscles tend to work in sympathy with each other. You cannot make your uterus contract but you can control your arms and legs, so we use these to produce 'mock' contractions. Contract the muscles of your right arm, breathe in, breathe out, and decontract or relax the whole of the rest of your body. Hold the contraction for about 20 seconds, paying particular attention to the relaxation of the left arm. Repeat, tightening your left arm and relaxing the rest of your body; then repeat, using alternate legs. Towards the end of your pregnancy when your abdomen becomes hard and your uterus is having a trial contraction, practise decontracting all the rest of your body and breathing steadily through the contraction.

Posture

Lying   If lying down causes breathlessness, dizziness, or bad heartburn, relief may be gained by lying on your side and being propped up from the waist, with pillows under your ribs, head, and shoulders. If the number of pillows under the head only is

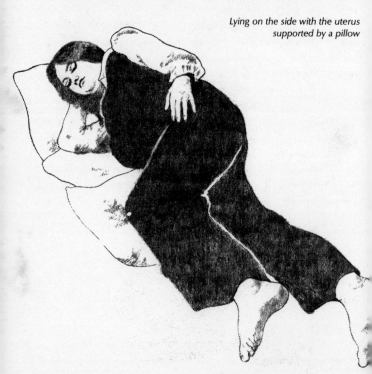

Lying on the side with the uterus
supported by a pillow

increased, a stiff neck may be added to your other problems! If your top hip aches, a small soft cushion may be put under the top knee, or under the bulge so that the uterus is supported in its correct position. On getting up, you should swing your legs over the side of the bed and sit on it for a few moments before you stand, so that you do not feel dizzy.

Kneeling   Kneeling may be an extremely comfortable position from which to watch television or read, but it is important not to sit back on your heels unless there is a thick cushion on them, so that pressure behind the knees is avoided. Squatting with the knees apart is another potentially dangerous position because of the strain exerted on the tissues between the legs which support the baby.

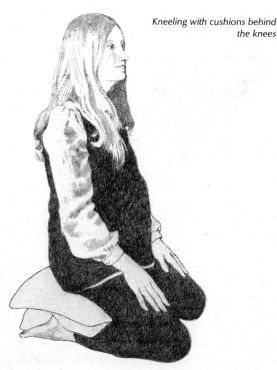

Kneeling with cushions behind the knees

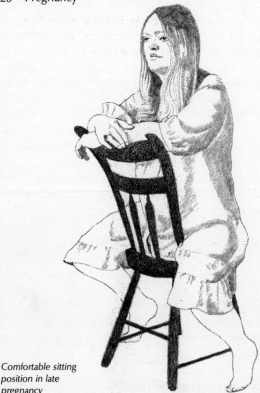

*Comfortable sitting
position in late
pregnancy*

Sitting   The bones of the spine must be supported properly, either by their own muscles or by cushions. The most comfortable positions are probably either sitting on a hard chair at a table, with your elbows resting on the table to lift your rib-cage and prevent excess pressure from the bulge on the lower ribs, or sitting on a narrow chair the wrong way round, your legs astride the seat, and your arms resting on the chair back. You could also try sitting on a low chair, such as a nursing chair, or on a soft, higher armchair with cushions behind your back, and your elbows supported on the chair arms. In a car, it is often most comfortable to sit on a cushion to prevent pressure in the groin area. When resting with the feet up, it is important to ensure that they are raised high enough – at least level with your bottom – and that there is no pressure in the groin.

Standing correctly

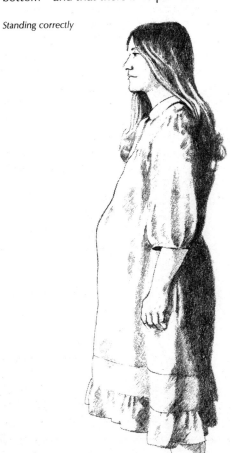

Standing and walking   Standing still should be avoided: the household chores should be done sitting or kneeling on a stool or the floor. When it is absolutely necessary to stand, keep the legs a little apart and take the body weight from one foot to the other. There is always a tendency to compensate for the extra weight of your baby by leaning back, either from your ankles or from the waist. As your figure changes you will find it necessary to guard against these tendencies, particularly when you are tired. Make yourself as tall as you can, pull your abdomen in slightly and tuck your 'tail' down as in the pelvic rocking exercise described above, and make sure that your weight is evenly balanced between the balls and heels of your feet. This posture should be maintained while walking. When shopping it is a good idea to check your reflection in plate-glass windows to make sure you are standing correctly – what feels right may not always look right.

Lifting   Stooping to lift a toddler, or a bag of shopping, can cause strain on the back. If you have a toddler, try to avoid lifting him, as far as possible. Teach him to climb safely in and out of his chair, and how to cope with the stairs. If he needs a cuddle, sit on a chair beside him, or kneel on the floor to bring yourself down to his level. If you have to carry a lot of shopping, always use two bags, one in each hand, to balance the weight, and when you pick them up, bend your knees or kneel on one knee, and use your legs to straighten up, not your back muscles.

Problems of pregnancy

The major physical characteristic of pregnancy is the swelling of your abdomen into what most mothers call their 'bulge' or 'bump'. However, other complex bodily changes are taking place which are not so obvious. Both the sheer size of the growing 'bump' and these other changes can cause discomforts, most of which can be alleviated in some way.

Care of your body

Relaxin, the relaxing hormone which is produced during pregnancy, affects all body structures. It loosens joints, so take care not to strain them. Activities such as walking, swimming, and dancing are very good but a programme of strenuous exercises is not advisable. It is very important to check your posture: that in itself is good exercise for your muscles.

The hormone also slows down the digestive and excretory systems, so eat smaller, more frequent meals and drink plenty of water, which helps to prevent constipation. Roughage is important – added bran in cereals and home baking, plus raw fruits and vegetables, help to prevent constipation. Eat at least one raw meal every day, such as a fruit or vegetable salad, and if constipation persists try taking a mixture of dried fruits and senna powder.

Relaxin slows the return circulation and can produce varicose veins. You can help to prevent these by doing some simple exercises whenever you have a few minutes to sit down – pull the feet up and down, circle them round, and make gripping movements with the toes. If necessary ask your doctor for a prescription for support hose – there are some which can be made to measure so that the length is correct for you. Wearing a lightweight pantie girdle during the last six to eight weeks of pregnancy supports the baby's weight when it has a considerable weight gain; it also helps to prevent overstretching of the abdomen and strain on the lower back, both of which tend to cause bad posture, and the resulting pressure makes varicose veins worse. (Vitamin E capsules can help to get rid of varicose veins. Ask your doctor about them.) If wearing a girdle seems a nuisance or bothers you, wear one when you are busy, and remove it when you are resting.

The rib-cage enlarges by 8–10 cm (3–4 inches) round its lower part towards the end of pregnancy and can cause backache, shoulder, and rib pain. To avoid this, your back should be straight – whether sitting, lying, standing, or kneeling.

Be careful about your posture when doing housework. Try sitting or kneeling on a stool at the sink instead of standing, sitting to prepare vegetables, kneeling to make the bed, and bending your knees rather than your back when you pick up objects from the floor. Try cleaning the bath when you are in it, instead of hanging over the side to do it.

Stretching both arms above your head for any length of time, lying flat on your back, having hot baths, and getting up too quickly from a lying or sitting position, can cause fainting. Sitting slumped in a chair may cause backache and indigestion, standing for too long increases the likelihood of varicose veins, and squatting with the legs apart exerts great pressure on the muscles at the base of the pelvis.

Dry, flaking, itching skin can be relieved by massaging in body lotion, almond oil, or other creams. When trying one you have not used before, put it on only a very small area of skin first in case it causes a rash. Itching may be relieved by using a lotion made by steeping nettle leaves in hot water and then letting the liquid cool before applying it. Stretch marks on the sides of the breasts may be reduced if you wear a sleep bra at night.

Minor ailments in pregnancy

catarrh	try a weak inhalation, garlic perles or sugar-coated garlic tablets, biochemic tissue salts (Combination Q).
bleeding gums	try massaging them with your finger-tips before brushing with a soft bristle brush.
indigestion	try eating smaller meals, sitting up very straight to eat them, and taking heartburn mixture (which works faster than tablets) *obtained on prescription from your doctor.*

backache	try correcting your posture, and wearing a light-weight girdle to support the weight of the baby, which eases sciatic and other similar pains.
piles	first cure any constipation; don't strain, and try a suppository of peeled garlic, retained overnight. Vitamin E may help.
swollen ankles	don't stand still; try sitting on a high chair, or on a cushion when in the car.
cramp	stretch the affected part, then quickly bend it; to avoid further attacks don't drink milk at bedtime, and stretch as you wake up with your heels down and toes up. Hip cramp may be relieved by taking your weight equally on both feet, especially when rising from a sitting position – say, from a chair or a car seat.
weight gain	with a correctly balanced diet and plenty of raw fruit and vegetables, wholewheat bread, and wholegrain cereals, weight gain should be normal.
stretch marks	cannot be prevented but may be kept to a minimum by keeping the skin supple (using cream or oil), correcting posture and having adequate support for the abdomen and breasts. Vitamin E oil may help remove scars.

varicose veins	avoid standing still, wearing tight garments, and being constipated.
aching feet	do foot exercises (circling the feet, pointing the toes, drawing up the toes as if picking up something under them), and avoid standing still for long periods.
feeling faint	avoid moving too quickly from a lying or sitting position, avoid smoky atmospheres and long journeys, and increase the iron intake in your diet.
itching (like thrush)	may be relieved by applying natural yoghurt to the vaginal area.
nausea/'morning sickness'	can occur at any time of day. See 'Diet in pregnancy' section for guidelines to alleviate it. Homoeopathic ipecac. may also help.
fatigue	may occur in early and late pregnancy and it is important not to force yourself to do too much. Alternate periods of rest and activity if you cannot have a daily rest lying down, and do not plan evening appointments which you cannot cancel.
abdominal or round ligament pain	pain below the 'bump', in the groins, is due to ligament strain and may be alleviated by wearing a lightweight pantie-girdle; resting with the feet up, with a pillow under the hips and under the head and shoulders; and taking great care over walking downstairs

and downhill (especially if holding a push-chair or shopping trolley).

pelvic discomfort   again, a lightweight girdle and correct posture will help, as will frequently repeated pelvic floor exercises (see p. 0).

vaginal discharge   is increased during pregnancy, but any offensive green, yellow, or bloodstained discharge should be reported to your doctor.

insomnia   having a small snack at bedtime, a warm bath, a hot water bottle, plenty of supporting pillows (see pp. 18–19), and cat-napping, assisted by relaxation and comfortably deep breathing, may all help.

contact lenses   it may be necessary to discontinue the use of these during pregnancy. If in doubt, consult your doctor.

bladder discomfort   the baby may appear to be rubbing his head on your bladder, causing soreness. 'Kneel-sitting' (see p. 19) on a pillow on your heels may relieve it.

Much interest is now being shown in the use of homoeopathic remedies. Two substances may be of help during pregnancy and labour: caulophyllum can improve the muscle tone of the uterus, and arnica tablets taken during and after labour may reduce bruising and make the pelvic floor area more comfortable. You may like to discuss this with your doctor. Further information can be obtained from The British Homoeopathic Assn., Basildon Court, 27a Devonshire Street, London W1N 1RJ.

Antenatal medical procedures

Whether you wish to have your baby at home or in hospital the pattern of antenatal medical care should be similar. Report to your doctor as soon as you think that you may be pregnant so that you can confirm the diagnosis and start planning for the birth of your baby. The sooner you do this, the better for your health and the baby's.

The first antenatal examination

During your first antenatal consultation the doctor or midwife will ask you questions about the details of any previous pregnancies, including miscarriages, abortions, previous births, and ectopic (tubal) pregnancies; your general state of health; how you feel now; past illnesses and operations; the medical history of your immediate family; any medicines or drugs that you may be taking; the date of your last menstrual period; details of your usual menstrual cycle, and what kind of contraception you were using until the time that you conceived.

The doctor will make a general physical examination: testing your urine, noting your weight, height, blood pressure and the state of your heart, lungs, breasts, and abdomen. If you have reached the third month (12 weeks) of your pregnancy, the doctor should be able to feel the top of your uterus just above the pubic bone at the front of your pelvis. If your pregnancy is less far advanced, enlargement, softening, and the change in the shape of your uterus characteristic of pregnancy can only be detected by feeling the uterus with two hands (bi-manual examination). This is done with one hand feeling through your abdominal wall and with one or two fingers of the other hand feeling the cervix and lower part of your uterus through the vagina. Such a bi-manual pelvic or vaginal examination also gives the doctor some idea of the shape and size of your pelvis, whether or not you have any fibroids (common benign non-cancerous tumours of the uterine muscle) or cysts on the ovaries that may cause problems, as well as confirming the

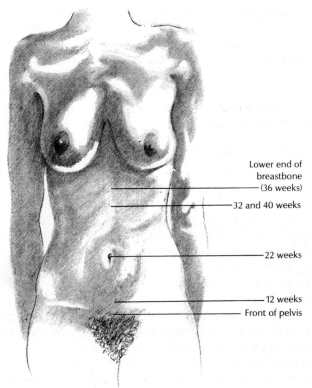

Lower end of
breastbone
(36 weeks)

32 and 40 weeks

22 weeks

12 weeks
Front of pelvis

Approximate height of uterus at different stages during pregnancy

diagnosis and duration of the pregnancy. At this time the doctor may also use a speculum (a metal instrument) to look into the vagina and see the cervix. This gives the doctor an opportunity to take a cytological smear from the cervix for the detection of any early pre-cancerous changes, and also to detect any infections such as 'thrush' (candida or monilia) or TV (*Trichomonas vaginitis*), which cause an irritating unpleasant-smelling discharge.

If the doctor cannot be sure that you are pregnant, it is simple to carry out a pregnancy test on your urine. In special circumstances, it is also possible to have a very sensitive pregnancy test done on your blood. If you are pregnant, this test will show positive within ten days of conception, whereas pregnancy tests on urine are unlikely to give a positive result until 14 days after you have missed a period.

A vaginal examination carried out gently in early pregnancy does not provoke miscarriage, but if you are worried about this tell your doctor before he makes the examination. The vaginal examination is helpful not only for the reasons given above, but to date the pregnancy, especially if you have a long or irregular menstrual cycle, and if you have just stopped taking oral contraceptives. A vaginal examination will be essential to detect an abnormal pregnancy in the uterus or in the tube.

Having completed the examination, the doctor should tell you his findings and give you his opinion as to how the pregnancy can be expected to proceed. Now is the time to discuss with the doctor where you will have your baby and who will look after you during pregnancy and labour (see 'The choice of birth at home', p. 91).

However you are to be cared for you may be given a Maternity Co-operation Card. You should carry this card with you whenever you have an examination. It contains a summary of your medical history, any tests carried out, and the progress of your pregnancy, so that the midwife or doctor who sees you has all the relevant information, and can then make his or her own notes.

Blood tests

At the time of your first antenatal examination, or soon afterwards, blood tests are carried out to identify your blood group; to determine whether or not your blood contains any antibodies (for example, the Rhesus negative factor) that could affect the baby; to assess the haemoglobin level and detect anaemia; to exclude syphilis; to find out whether you are susceptible or resistant (immune) to German measles (rubella); and, if you come from Africa, Asia, or a Mediterranean country, to check whether your blood has any unusual haemoglobin (sickle cell test) which makes the red blood cells more fragile and causes anaemia.

Blood tests to estimate haemoglobin levels and detect any antibody formation are usually repeated later in pregnancy at 28 weeks and again at 36 weeks.

Antenatal visits throughout pregnancy

During a normal pregnancy the doctor or midwife will ask to see you every four weeks from the first visit until 28 weeks, every two weeks from 28 weeks to 36 weeks, and then every week until the baby is born. If any abnormality is detected, or if you need special care, you may be asked to attend the antenatal clinic more frequently than this.

At each visit you will be asked how you feel. You will be weighed and have your blood pressure taken, and your urine will be checked to make sure that there are no signs of problems. Your abdomen will be examined to see how the uterus is growing and later on how the baby is lying. If you are expecting a first baby, you will usually feel the baby move for the first time between 18 and 22 weeks. If you have had a baby before, you may feel it move for the first time as early as 16 weeks. The baby's heart can usually be heard with an ordinary foetal stethoscope at about 24 weeks. It can be heard much earlier than this, even before you are able to feel the baby's movements, if ultrasound is used to detect the beating heart.

Tests of foetal health and placental function

In a normal pregnancy with a healthy baby this is most easily measured by the steady increase in your weight, the quality and strength of the baby's movements, and the growth rate of your uterus. In some women the rate of growth of the pregnancy, and/or complicating medical conditions (such as high blood pressure, diabetes, previous stillbirths, premature deliveries, and trouble with the baby after birth) may cause concern. In such circumstances it may be desirable to follow the baby's progress as closely as possible to decide whether or not early delivery, perhaps by Caesarean section, might be in the baby's best interests. This can be done by repeated ultrasound measurement of the baby's head; repeated tests on your blood to measure the level of hormones such as oestrogen and HPL (human placental lactogen); repeated measurements in 24-hour collections of urine of the amount of oestrogens; recording the baby's heart-rate to see whether or not the pattern of activity and variation is normal, which is a guide to the state of the oxygen supply to the baby.

Estimation of pelvic shape and size

One of the aims of antenatal care is to detect any hindrance which might arise if the baby should be too big to pass through the pelvic bones and the birth canal. This is called cephalo-pelvic disproportion. In a healthy woman of normal height this is most unlikely; however, in women who are shorter than average the pelvic bones may be too small, and this may cause delay and difficulty in labour. In women expecting a first baby, the head usually settles into the pelvic cavity (engages) some time after 36 weeks and before labour begins. In a woman who has had one or more babies before, engagement of the head may not occur until labour starts. Her previous experience will be a guide to the width of her pelvis and the length and difficulty of labour she may expect.

Many doctors do another routine pelvic examination during the last four weeks of pregnancy to make a clinical estimate of the shape and size of your pelvis in relation to the size of the baby's head. In a few women it may be necessary to find out much more about the pelvic shape and size from an X-ray. This may be suggested if you are very small, if the baby is thought to be very large, if the baby's head does not engage easily, or if you expect a breech delivery (see p. 109). Usually only one film is taken with you standing sideways on to the X-ray film with a ruler between your legs, so that the size of the pelvic outlet, cavity, and inlet can be measured directly from the film.

Ultrasonic examination

Using a source of very high frequency sound that cannot be heard by the human ear (ultrasound), it is possible to examine the contents of the uterus in pregnancy by plotting on a television screen how the ultrasound signals are reflected back from various surfaces such as the wall of the uterus, the placenta, the baby, and his beating heart. By measuring the size of the baby's head the duration of pregnancy can be established. If these measurements are repeated the growth rate of the baby can be followed. The measurements usually made are of the baby's head size between the two bony prominences above the ears. Using ultrasound, the movements of the baby's heart can be detected before they can be heard, the situation of the placenta can be located, and if twins are present they can be detected. Some obstetricians ask every woman to have three ultrasound scans to measure the baby's growth rate so that the duration of pregnancy can be known as accurately as possible. Other obstetricians are more selective and only use ultrasound scans to obtain further information for special reasons, such as before amniocentesis; if more than one baby is suspected; if foetal death is suspected; if the growth rate of the baby is either too fast or too slow; if the menstrual dates are doubtful and there is a need to estimate the expected date of delivery more accurately; or, if there has been bleeding and it is necessary to know whether the placenta is attached low down in the uterus (placenta praevia).

There is no evidence that exposure of babies to ultrasound is harmful, but on the other hand there is no absolute proof that it is harmless. Those using ultrasound can misinterpret what is seen. Therefore some consultants believe that ultrasound is best used selectively for particular reasons, and that the scans should not be used as the only basis on which to make decisions.

Detection of congenital abnormalities before birth

About one in forty babies born alive has some physical defect.

Most are minor, such as birthmarks, but some are serious, and a few do not allow the baby to survive or lead a normal independent life. Not all abnormalities can be detected before birth, particularly those of the heart and major blood vessels, and those of the limbs and digestive system.

If it is suspected that your baby may be at risk, special tests can be carried out to confirm or refute the possibility. Most of these tests involve a procedure called amniocentesis (see below).

At present, if an abnormal baby is detected in pregnancy, nothing can be done to correct the deformity. The aim of detecting abnormal pregnancies is, therefore, to offer those concerned the opportunity of considering whether to continue with the pregnancy, or to have it terminated. If this is not a choice you would wish to consider, there is no point in having the tests carried out.

Amniocentesis   This is the method used to obtain a sample of the amniotic fluid surrounding the baby. A local anaesthetic solution is injected to numb a small part of the mother's abdominal wall just below the umbilicus (navel). A needle is pushed through the numb part into the uterus taking care to avoid the placenta so that a small sample of the baby's amniotic fluid can be sucked out with a syringe for examination in the laboratory.

Neural tube defects   The commonest of the more serious defects (one in 200 births) involves the development of the spinal cord, spinal column, the brain, and the skull – so-called neural tube defects, which include spina bifida and anencephaly. Neural tube defects can be detected by testing the mother's blood between 16 and 22 weeks of pregnancy for alfa-fetoprotein. If this is present in larger amounts than usual, it merely suggests that the baby may have a neural tube defect, but it is not conclusive evidence that this is so unless alfa-fetoproetin is also found in abnormal quantities in the water (amniotic fluid) surrounding the baby. The alfa-fetoprotein level of the mother's blood is also raised with a normal twin pregnancy or if the baby has died; it also rises as pregnancy progresses. Therefore, no attempt is usually made to obtain amniotic fluid for testing until the duration of the pregnancy has been checked and the possibility of twins has been excluded. This can most easily be done by ultrasound examination (see above), when the situation of the placenta (afterbirth) can also be located.

Down's syndrome (mongolism)   This is another abnormality that can be detected in pregnancy before the baby is born. Down's syndrome is caused by an abnormality in the baby's chromosomes, which store the genes, or blueprints for the structure and function of our cells. To detect or exclude Down's syndrome, the chromosome constitution of the baby is ascertained before it is born. Fluid obtained by amniocentesis will contain living cells shed from the baby's skin which can be isolated in the laboratory and grown in tissue culture. About three to four weeks later, when the cells divide, the chromosome pattern can be recognised. The tests required naturally cause anxiety, because they cannot be completed quickly and it is not usually possible to obtain water from around the baby by amniocentesis before 16 weeks. This means you will not know the answer until about 20 to 22 weeks of pregnancy. The abnormal chromosomes of mongolism may be passed on to the baby if either parent is carrying this defect, or more commonly if the ovum (egg) is abnormal before it is fertilised, which is more likely to happen in women who become pregnant in later life.

Other abnormalities   A few other rare abnormalities can be detected by tests on the amniotic fluid (e.g. Thalassaemia, an inherited abnormal haemoglobin causing anaemia). Tests on amniotic fluid can also be made on Rhesus negative women with antibodies to find out the best time for delivery, and whether or not the baby needs a transfusion in the uterus before birth. Amniotic fluid obtained by amniocentesis in late pregnancy (after 28 weeks) is also used to determine the maturity of the baby, particularly of his lungs, to know – if premature delivery is indicated – how well the baby is likely to be able to expand his lungs and breathe on his own.

Ask for explanations

Throughout your pregnancy you are entitled to know, and you should know, what is happening, why tests are necessary, and what the results are. At no time in pregnancy should anything be done to you unless you have received a full explanation which you have understood and willingly accepted. If you do not understand, ask for an explanation. If you are afraid of the tests in any way, say so. If you are not given an explanation that satisfies you, go on asking questions until you are satisfied. If necessary, enlist the aid of your partner. Antenatal care, unfortunately, easily becomes a mechanical and impersonal process for many doctors and midwives, unless you are prepared to question them and make it necessary for them to treat you as an individual. Make them aware tactfully that it is your baby, and that your fears and doubts may be as important as the results of any tests that are carried out.

Diet during pregnancy

It is not usually necessary to change your eating habits completely because you are pregnant, but you may wish to take a look at your diet to see if it can be improved. To remain healthy, you should eat a balanced nutritious diet, as varied as you can possibly make it. Adjusting your diet can help alleviate some of the discomforts associated with pregnancy.

Sources of essential nutrients

Eat sensibly from the following groups of foods daily, and avoid eating too much of any one food or group.
Protein   Meat, liver, kidneys, poultry, fish, fish roe; cheese, milk, eggs, cottage cheese, yoghurt; peas, beans, lentils, soya

beans, peanuts; wheatgerm, brown rice, whole barley; sesame and sunflower seeds; avocado pears, brussels sprouts, spinach; bread.

Carbohydrates   Flour, bread, breakfast cereals; root vegetables, peas, potatoes, bananas; sugar, honey, syrup, treacle and all confectionery; soft drinks, alcohol; milk.

Fats   Meat, sausages and processed meats, poultry, herrings, pilchards, sardines, sprats; butter, cheese, milk, eggs; oils, margarine, lard; nuts.

Calcium   Cheese, milk, yoghurt, eggs; bread (wholemeal and white), oatmeal, stoneground flour, soya; nuts, sesame seeds; treacle; fish; oranges, raspberries, blackberries, dried fruit; spinach, broccoli, cabbage, swedes, turnips, cauliflower.

Iron   Meat, kidneys, heart, liver; cereals, bread, flour, wheatgerm, breakfast cereal, soya; eggs; pilchards, sardines; dried fruit; haricot and butter beans, lentils; spinach, parsley, watercress; cocoa, chocolate; black treacle; nuts.

Vitamin A   Butter, cheese, eggs, milk; fish liver oils, margarine, oily fish; liver, heart, kidneys; carrots, apricots, tomatoes, green vegetables (especially spinach and watercress).

B vitamins   Wheatgerm, whole grains; liver; brewer's yeast, wholewheat (wheatgerm) bread.

Vitamin C   Citrus fruits, berry fruits; green vegetables, especially raw and salad vegetables, green and red peppers, potatoes; drinks made from blackcurrants, oranges, or rosehips.

Vitamin D   Fish liver oils, margarine, oily fish; eggs, butter, cheese, liver. Vitamin D is also manufactured by the skin in the presence of sunlight, so try to get out of doors on sunny days.

Additional advice for a wholesome diet

Avoid sugar and the artificial additives, colourings and flavourings found in abundance in convenience foods and bottled drinks and squashes. Remember that wholewheat flour and wholegrain cereals are more nutritious than highly processed ones. Ask your baker specifically for wholewheat bread, rather than simply 'brown' bread, which is not necessarily the same.

Many fresh fruits and vegetables are higher in food value and generally lower in cost than processed ones. Vegetables and fruits are more nutritious eaten raw. Vitamin C, particularly, is destroyed by excess heat and prolonged exposure to air. To cook vegetables, steam or boil them as briefly as possible in very little water to avoid the loss of too many vitamins and minerals. Green vegetables should be shredded finely and cooked for not more than three minutes. If they smell stale they have been overcooked and contain little nourishment.

Advice to vegetarians and vegans

Anyone cutting out meat and fish from the diet can obtain adequate protein from other sources (cheese, soya products). Be sure to eat a variety of foods at each meal, in order to combine the elements that make up a complete diet.

If, as a vegan, you also avoid dairy products, be particularly careful to obtain essential nutrients by eating unrefined foods, plenty of green vegetables, dried prunes, and apricots. Complete vitamin B formula is advisable as a vitamin supplement.

For further information contact:

The Vegetarian Society, Parkdale, Durham Road, Altrincham, Cheshire.

The London Vegetarian Centre, 53 Marloes Road, London W8 6ID.

The Vegan Society, 47 Highlands Road, Leatherhead, Surrey.

Suggested changes to your diet during pregnancy

What changes should you make to your diet when you become pregnant?

You should eat adequate food containing protein during pregnancy. Protein builds the tissue which forms your baby, a solid placenta, and a strong uterus. Protein in the diet keeps the blood sugar level high, which in turn helps prevent nausea and depression.

Your calcium intake should be increased, since it is necessary for the development of the bones and teeth (both milk teeth and permanent ones) of the foetus. Teeth begin to form at four to six weeks after conception.

Iron intake should also be increased. Your doctor may prescribe additional iron and folic acid in the form of tablets, to ensure that you do not become anaemic and run-down. Iron-containing foods should be included in your diet too, particularly if you react adversely to iron tablets.

Vitamin A consumption should be increased, since it is responsible for building up your resistance to infection, has a vital function in vision, and can help prevent or relieve allergies and acne.

The B vitamins help to eradicate skin problems, nervousness, constipation, lack of energy, and increase the production of milk.

You should also take more vitamin C. It is involved in the absorption of iron, in keeping tissues strong and healthy, in detoxifying the body, and building a strong placenta.

Vitamin D is required to help the body absorb calcium and phosphorus.

Vitamin E supplement may help to retain the pregnancy and to improve circulation, can treat varicose veins and piles, and may help in the production of hormones. It is destroyed by iron, so you should avoid taking the two together. Leave a gap of about 12 hours between them, taking one in the morning and the other at night.

Coping with problems during pregnancy

Weight   Your doctor will keep careful track of your weight gain. It is important to eat well when you are pregnant. During pregnancy the body's metabolism changes and fat is put on very easily to help lactation when the baby is born. While there is no sense in starving yourself, there is also no sense in gorging just because you are going to put on weight anyway! Most women put on around 13 kg (2 stones) when they are pregnant and find that they are 3–6 kg (7–14 lb) heavier after giving birth than before they became pregnant.

If you are worried about weight gain, cut down on fats and carbohydrates, and eat fresh fruit and vegetables rather than biscuits and cakes. If you cannot go without sugar in tea or coffee, limit your intake and find an alternative such as water, fresh fruit juice, meat or yeast extract, or herb tea.

Nausea and sickness   Many pregnant women suffer from nausea especially during the early months. There seems to be no certain cure for this, but it may help to eat frequently, or to have a snack before rising. Some people find bread and butter or something sweet relieves the symptoms, others find dry toast or cracker biscuits help. If nausea or sickness is really troublesome or persistent, ask your doctor to prescribe something for you.

Indigestion and heartburn   These conditions can also be a nuisance in pregnancy, but they are not inevitable. The first thing to do is to eat regularly, avoid large meals or going too long without food, and not to eat foods which you know will cause heartburn. If the problem persists, go to your doctor. If the first thing doesn't work, try something else. You may find that milk of magnesia mixture acts much quicker than tablets.

Constipation   This is another annoying problem in pregnancy, but it can be lessened by eating foods with a high fibre content. Eat wholewheat rather than white bread, and try baking with wholewheat flour. Try breakfast cereals, like muesli (avoiding the manufactured ones with added sugar), with a lot of wholemeal and bran in them. Make sure that you eat plenty of vegetables, fresh fruit, prunes, and figs.

Other advice during pregnancy

In general, follow your own appetite, but in moderation. You may find yourself craving new foods during this time of change in the body's chemistry. Take advantage of this but try to vary your diet as much as possible.

Spirits and other alcoholic drinks should be taken only in moderation, as alcohol crosses the placenta and may affect the baby adversely.

Stop smoking. It is known to reduce the size of your baby, and therefore his chances of survival.

Take special care of your teeth. Pregnancy gingivitis can be avoided by regular, systematic brushing with a soft-bristled toothbrush and by cutting down on sugar. Tooth decay is caused by maternal neglect, not by the baby's calcium needs.

Sex in pregnancy

It is only recently that people have felt free to talk about enjoying love-making during pregnancy; before then it was a curiously forbidden subject. It was obvious that the prospective parents had made love in order to conceive their baby, but after that they were expected to develop only maternal and paternal feelings and to sublimate any sexual passion. It was hinted that sex could even damage the baby in some undefined way. The fact that mothers and fathers are also lovers was glossed over.

Nowadays light is being shed on this taboo. It has its origins deep in history when, for instance, hunters, fishermen, or warriors were expected to abstain from sex before important ventures; when pregnant women were thought of as unclean and threatening, or so sacred that they were inviolable. It was also believed that pregnant women were in a state of transition between maidenhood and motherhood and were thus vulnerable. These superstitious feelings sometimes manifest themselves today in areas where good luck must be courted – many sportsmen abstain from sex before important competitions in that belief that this will somehow conserve their strength and not 'waste vital forces' in ejaculation. And many couples feel that there is something morally wrong or physically risky in making love freely and happily during pregnancy. This is sad because pregnancy is a time when loving partners feel especially tender towards one another. For those who normally rely on the cap or the sheath for contraception, there is the joy of spontaneous lovemaking.

Avoiding miscarriage

There may be good reasons for avoiding intercourse at certain times if you have a history of miscarriage and your doctor advises it. You can devise together other ways of making love during each week when a period would have been due during the first three months, if you have already lost one baby early in pregnancy.

It is not the penis in the vagina which can cause miscarriage, but the woman's own orgasm. Orgasm causes about five to ten contractions of the uterus which may set off other contractions. If the baby is ready to be born, or miscarried, these contractions may initiate labour. On the other hand, if your baby is overdue, an orgasm may induce it to arrive – far more pleasantly than a drip or cervical sweep!

A relaxed attitude

Sometimes a pregnant woman feels she must concentrate on protecting the unborn child at all costs, treating herself as some fragile object which will disintegrate at the first knock. It is much more healthy to be relaxed and happy about sex, and life in general during pregnancy. Affectionate, tender, and spontaneous lovemaking, and the total release of orgasm, will show couples how naturally they can achieve relaxation. Many people, contemplating antenatal courses which teach relaxation exercises, feel that there is some special athleticism involved and doubt the ability of their own bodies to achieve this state: in fact, complete relaxation in a labour which is going well is, for many women, very much like relaxation after lovemaking when one feels release, calm, and emotional warmth. After the culmination of a satisfying labour and delivery women can experience an emotional 'high' akin to the deep peace which follows the most moving orgasm. The look a man sees on his wife's face after orgasm may also be there when she is enjoying her labour – her skin glows, her cheeks are flushed, her eyes shine, her hair is damp and untidy, and they both have a sense of deep satisfaction. Lovemaking and birth are both experiences which focus our attention upon the quiet centre in ourselves – and both can be upset by inhibitions or outside distractions.

Lack of interest in sex

Some couples find they are more interested in sex during the wife's pregnancy. However, some women may be temporarily revolted by the idea of sex, unaroused by things which they usually find pleasurable, or frustratingly unable to reach a climax. You should both remember to be patient if this happens and try other ways of showing your love. Many of us do the same mutually satisfying things for years on end and it is a stimulating challenge to have to try new techniques.

Husbands need loving reassurance and demonstrative sympathy – cuddling, caressing, humour, and passion. Often a man may feel isolated from his wife's pregnancy, or jealous of the coming child, and envious of his wife's ability to nurture new life within her.

Whatever temporary problems you may have, don't take your mutual love for granted: express it again and again.

Adjustments

The pregnant woman has to make enormous mental and physical adjustments during the first three months. She will be conscious of bodily changes outside her control, perhaps including nausea and vomiting, and may feel that her person-ality is changing in ways she cannot understand. She may have mixed feelings about her pregnant body, and will not yet have had the excitement and reassurance of feeling her baby move inside her. She may be afraid to tell people she is pregnant, and may find it odd that although so much is happening inside her, there is so little to show for it. She may enjoy sex more than ever; on the other hand, she may find it distasteful.

The middle three months tend to be the most emotionally stable for the pregnant woman. As she watches her abdomen enlarge, however, she may worry that she will eventually be so large that her husband will find her unattractive. At this point it is as well to remember that growth of girth in pregnancy is gradual, and that you will not be slim one day and enormous the next! There is time for both of you to acclimatize to your changing shape.

In the last three months the woman may be physically tired from the weight of her uterus and uncomfortable from its bulk, sleepless because of the baby's movements, suffering from heartburn, anxiously looking forward to the birth, and dismayed by the vastly pregnant figure she has become. Sex may be the last thing on her mind. In spite of this, she may find that her body is exquisitely sensitive to gentle caressing and that once she has allowed herself to become in the mood, she is more responsive than ever.

At other times the woman may find she cannot concentrate on sex, becomes bored with it, or fails to go along with her body's urgings. Sex manuals emphasize it so much that it can seem heretical to say that one can cope without simultaneous orgasm for a time, but this can be a satisfactory solution for some couples. You should discuss such difficulties with your husband to avoid any misunderstandings.

Sometimes a woman goes through the whole of her pregnancy guarding the unborn child as though her husband were attacking and defiling it. This can happen because she believes sex is unclean, or because she is so hungry for a baby that she will not share it – or herself – with her husband. This may indicate a serious long-term problem for the marriage. Help with the difficulty requires counselling from a marriage guidance expert.

Positions

The sheer physical changes caused by pregnancy mean that a couple will need to adapt their sexual technique. The 'missionary position' with the man on top, is very uncomfortable for a pregnant woman with a bulging abdomen and sensitive, full breasts. It can be achieved with the aid of pillows under her head and shoulders but may still induce heartburn and discomfort from deep penetration. (It is a good idea to buy extra pillows for use during lovemaking in pregnancy and for support during breastfeeding afterwards.)

The pregnant woman may find her extra-sensitive breasts an unexpected bonus, since they will be particularly responsive to her husband's touch and oral caresses. Indeed, this is a most pleasurable and effective way of preparing the nipples for breastfeeding (see p. 56).

Try side-to-side positions with the woman supported by pillows if her abdomen is very large. She can also kneel astride her sitting husband so that she can control the depth of penetration and he can stimulate her breasts at the same time. When the baby's head is engaged, the wife can try kneeling, crouching or lying so that her husband enters her vagina from behind. The uterus will then be virtually free from pressure since it lies almost at right angles to the vagina.

If pregnancy is advanced it may be more comfortable for the woman if her husband departs from the classic ideal of ejaculating after, or during, her orgasm. There may not be enough room in the tissues of the pelvic floor for her to contain the erect penis and also do the necessary pelvic thrusts which culminate in her orgasm. Experiment with the husband ejaculating first and then bringing his wife to orgasm afterwards.

Emotional preparation for parenthood

Pregnancy is a perfectly normal state for a woman to be in, but it is also a time of mental and physical adjustment, just like any other major change in your life. Your emotional responses to the pregnancy are just as important as the physical changes you are experiencing: you may, for instance, become suddenly aware of all the responsibility you have taken on, not only for the development of your baby before it is born, but also for the care and raising of a child which will be dependent on you for many years to come. Or you may find yourself swamped by such variety of advice and such a mass of choices that you do not know where to turn, because what seemed so simple – to have a baby – now involves all kinds of uncertainties you had not anticipated. Fortunately the nine months of gestation give you plenty of time in which to prepare to be a parent – it doesn't happen overnight. And it may be comforting to remind yourself that the baby will also be a first-timer and will not be comparing your efforts at parenting with anyone else's!

Pregnancies are very different experiences for different people. Some people are delighted to be pregnant, others are not pleased at all, still others accept the situation without great emotion either way. Some women find that pregnancy makes them feel unwell or ungainly, other women feel that they have never been healthier, and yet others cope with some discomforts and inconveniences but enjoy some benefits as well. Some couples find that pregnancy is a welcome and positive extension of their marriage; others find it a strain on their relationship, whether or not the baby was planned. Your pregnancy will be unlike anyone else's and will depend more on your personality than on anyone else's experience. It is best to take your pregnancy as it comes, neither counting on storybook bliss nor expecting the worst to happen.

When you do have bad days – and they come to virtually everyone at some point – try to find something really enjoyable to do as compensation and don't let yourself be led into thinking that the discouragement or discomfort will necessarily continue or that there is no solution. Treating yourself to whatever seems a self-indulgent pleasure in the circumstances will often have a restorative effect: if you are at home, put the chores aside and curl up in an armchair to read, do some fancy cooking, go for a walk, or invite a neighbour in for a cup of coffee; if you are at work, look forward to a long lazy bath when you reach home, have something special for lunch, get some fresh air during a break, or have a cup of tea (special flavoured teas and herbal teas may be particularly refreshing). If you feel like it, decide on the spur of the moment to do something special with your husband – maybe there is a film you have been wanting to see – or, on the other hand, allow yourself to decline invitations if you feel too tired to socialize.

When a pregnancy is confirmed, a woman's body suddenly becomes the subject of unblushing attention, with everyone – doctor and midwife, colleagues, family, and neighbours – talking freely about how well or tired she is looking, what and how much she should or should not eat, how big or how small her abdomen is, what exercise she should or should not take, and so forth. The feeling that the pregnancy which you thought was a private and loving affair between you and your husband is now a matter for public discussion can be very upsetting, and it is easy to resent the feeling that people seem to treat you as if you no longer had any interests other than the baby and indeed were important only because of the baby. Even if you faithfully attend your regular antenatal checks, and recognize their importance in ensuring your health and the baby's, you may feel that all this attention invades your privacy, questions your ability to take care of yourself, and implies that your body is no longer your own but belongs to the clinic, or the doctor, or the baby, more than to yourself.

Pregnancy involves so many changes that is not surprising that it takes some time to adjust to the idea. Just as starting a new job often raises doubts about whether you have made the right choice until you have settled in, so starting a family may give you some second thoughts. This is perfectly natural. At some point in pregnancy practically every woman wishes she had never embarked on the adventure. For most, this is only a temporary feeling, but for some it lasts throughout the pregnancy and colours the entire experience.

The woman who resents pregnancy

Some women simply do not like being pregnant. It may be that pregnancy makes the woman feel physically unwell, although she wants the baby, or it may be that she really does not want to have a baby at all, for whatever reason: perhaps she had planned a career which just does not fit in with being a mother; perhaps her personal circumstances have changed so that she wishes she had never become pregnant; perhaps the pregnancy was unplanned and came as an unwanted upset to the couple's expectations. If she has always been super-efficient she may hate the forgetfulness that so often comes with pregnancy; if she is accustomed to subduing her body to her intellectual needs or to pressures of work she may resent the tiredness and digestive demands of pregnancy; if she has led an active social life she may dread that pregnancy will make her feel or be unattractive and that having a baby will put an end to her freedom.

When a woman like this first realizes that she is pregnant, she may become extremely depressed and consider abortion, or she may refuse to accept that she is pregnant, but as time passes and her labour seems far ahead she may get used to the idea. When her 'bump' starts to show she may go through another bad patch – perhaps wearing a tight girdle to flatten her abdomen or starving herself in the hope that if she becomes thin she will not look pregnant. Perhaps the worst time is when she finally gives up work and begins to feel trapped at home. Her antenatal appointments become more frequent, she is offered antenatal classes, and everyone around her not only seems to be conspiring to remind her that soon she will be a mother, but also assumes that she is delighted at the prospect. She may easily decide to opt out of experiencing her labour by requesting an induction-and-epidural package, letting the machines and the doctor do everything so that she is minimally involved. (Of course, not every woman who seeks the help of medical technology during childbirth is 'opting out' – sometimes a woman will need an epidural to make her birth safer.)

This is painting the blackest picture and no one person is likely to go through all these negative stages; but it would be unrealistic and unwise to pretend that pregnancy automatically brings bliss, or that motherhood automatically means joy. Dreamy fantasies portrayed in advertisements bear little relation to the way most people feel and live.

To counteract these gloomy possibilities the frustrated career woman needs to use her intellect to make a career out of her pregnancy and motherhood. You may find comfort during your pregnancy by enquiring into the chances of either taking the baby to work with you or finding a registered baby-minder. The same applies of course to the woman who needs to work for financial reasons. If your job is not physically demanding, you may be able to continue with your work throughout your pregnancy. If you feel forced by the pressures of your family or neighbours to stay at home with your baby, this could have an adverse effect on your feelings towards the child; it is far better to find some way of returning to a job if that is what *you* need to do and then you may be able to be your own kind of 'good mother' and enjoy your child during the times between work. However, it is important that the baby has a constant caretaker and is not passed around to just any willing person.

The local county social services department is a good source of information about registered child-minders. For information about financial allowances you should consult the Department of Health and Social Security.

The changing hormone pattern during pregnancy can be a cause of mood swings, but they are not an excuse for constant bad temper and general dissatisfaction. Set about coping with pregnancy in a sensible manner: inform yourself about aspects of pregnancy, labour, and motherhood – and in particular take care of your diet. If you eat correctly you should feel and look well, the minor ills of pregnancy will be minimized, and the baby's growth and development will be helped.

Further observations

So far we have considered the difficulties of the woman who wishes she were not pregnant, but even the woman who is overjoyed to find herself pregnant may have problems. You may have periods of excessive tiredness, of feeling sick, of apparently unaccountable depression or anxiety. If you are eating correctly and getting an adequate amount of rest and exercise but still feeling low, you may like to add a vitamin E supplement to your diet. This will help the hormone balance and improve the condition of the placenta. The woman who becomes severely depressed or who habitually miscarries about the third to fourth month of pregnancy may be helped by progesterone therapy prescribed by her doctor. This usually involves a course of injections. Some women feel well if they take extra iron and vitamin B. In all of these cases, however, consult your doctor.

The woman who is fit and happy during her pregnancy is likely to transmit her confidence and well being to her husband so that he may share with her the joyful reality of pregnancy and anticipation of parenthood. She is likely to glow with health, to be keen to work with her body in adapting to pregnancy and coping with labour, and to be excited at the prospect of seeing her own baby.

Pregnancy can be a trying time for an expectant father, who may have just as many anxieties as his wife. Will the baby be normal? Might I lose my job and not be able to support my wife and child financially? If my wife becomes depressed during pregnancy will she ever return to normal? And so on. The man and woman may need to reassure and support each other. It is a good idea for *both* parents to inform themselves about the baby's growth and development and what happens to the mother during pregnancy, and the same applies to labour and parenthood. If you have anxieties which cannot be cleared up in antenatal classes or by reading, you could go together to the antenatal clinic so that there are two of you to ask the questions, and to make sure that you see a sufficiently senior member of the staff until you have answers which satisfy and reassure you. Discuss beforehand the gist of what you want to say and what you want to find out, and remember that should a choice be necessary, you can go away to discuss the matter by yourselves and return later to the doctor to let him know your decision. It is likely to be difficult to talk with the doctor if you are lying undressed on the examination couch, so ask the doctor if you can see him again when you are dressed to discuss his recommendations.

Nowadays men and women are able to choose when and if they will have children, and this makes it a natural step for them to want to take responsibility for the health of the mother and the baby during pregnancy and to give the baby as well-prepared and gentle a birth as possible.

The advantages of breastfeeding

One of the things you and your husband should think about before your baby is born is whether you want to breastfeed. Breastfeeding is so good for the baby that you should consider giving it a try at least – and at best plan to breastfeed for as long as you can.

Most breastfeeding failures arise from lack of information. There are many myths about breastfeeding, and there are also many facts which you can learn beforehand about the advantages of natural feeding and about how your breasts function. In this way you will understand what is happening and will be able to differentiate between good and bad advice. It will also give you calmness and self-confidence, which are very important.

Breastfeeding is becoming fashionable again after a time when bottle-feeding was the norm. This is good, but it can mean that in many places nurses and midwives trained during an era when artificial feeding predominated are not used to giving breastfeeding help and may pay lip service to it while unintentionally giving inaccurate advice. So learn enough during pregnancy to be your own counsel when the baby arrives. Of course, if problems occur that you cannot cope with, you can always get in touch with your doctor, your health visitor, or your local NCT breastfeeding counsellor, who has been trained by the Breastfeeding Promotion Group of the NCT to give advice on practical, non-medical, breastfeeding problems.

Some good reasons for breastfeeding

Midwives and doctors agree that breast milk is the perfect first food for babies. Its constituents are quite different in their proportions from cows' milk, which has to be extensively modified in order to make it suitable for human babies. It is more difficult for the kidneys of young babies to excrete the extra mineral salts found in artificial milks.

Colostrum, the high-protein fluid which precedes breast milk proper, is particularly valuable. It contains antibodies to many of the diseases you have had or have been immunized against and helps protect against the bacteria which cause gastro-enteritis. The risk of gastro-enteritis is much greater in bottle-fed babies, especially where bottle sterilization is inefficient.

There is a certain amount of evidence that breastfed babies seem less likely to develop allergies such as eczema and asthma.

Breastfed babies are less likely to get fat than bottle-fed babies. Fat babies often become fat adults, and fat adults are more prone to heart disease, arterial disease, and diabetes. Fat babies are also more prone to colds and chest infections.

Breastfed babies are never constipated. Although they sometimes go for several days without a bowel motion, because breast milk is so perfectly absorbed, the stool – when it comes – is always soft. Breastfed babies' motions have a less strong smell than those produced by bottle-fed babies, because there are different fats in breast milk.

Breastfeeding helps you to get your figure back to normal more quickly. Soon after birth the hormones involved in breast feeding cause 'afterpains' which help the uterus to contract back to its pre-pregnancy size and position. A longer period of breastfeeding uses up any extra fat which has been put on in pregnancy (for just this purpose).

Breastfeeding saves time – a valuable commodity to the new mother. Breast milk is always available, at the right temperature, when your baby is hungry. He never has to be kept waiting while you sterilize bottles or warm up feeds.

Breastfeeding is cheaper than bottle-feeding: bottles, teats, sterilizing equipment, and artificial milk all cost money. However, a breastfeeding mother needs more food for herself than a woman who is feeding her baby artificially. She will probably want to have a bottle and sterilizing solution available for emergencies.

Breastfeeding gives you automatic closeness to your baby. For the child, it is warmth, comfort, and food all rolled into one. For you, the mother, it is usually a very enjoyable experience.

Breast milk is a complete food for your baby for the first four to six months of life. Since the risks of ill-health are greater when the baby is very young, breastfeeding for even as little as two weeks is an advantage.

How the breasts produce milk

You will be more confident of your ability to breastfeed if you know a little about how your breasts work. The shape and size of your breasts does not affect your success in breastfeeding: large breasts do not indicate a plentiful milk supply, any more than small breasts mean a limited one. Breastfeeding is part of the reproductive cycle. Both conception and birth set hormones in action which cause changes to take place in the breasts in preparation for feeding your baby.

Pregnancy　Tenderness or tingling of the breasts and nipples are among the earliest signs of pregnancy. Milk glands replace the fat in your breasts, causing them to get bigger. The nipples and the pigmented area around them, the areola, enlarge and darken. This may be more noticeable if you have dark hair or

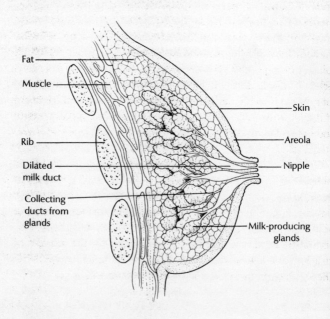

Fat

Muscle

Rib

Dilated
milk duct

Collecting
ducts from
glands

Skin

Areola

Nipple

Milk-producing
glands

The breast, showing where milk is produced

dark skin. The breasts start to make a sticky, yellow fluid, called colostrum, which may leak, forming crusts on the nipple.

After birth   For the first few days the breasts make colostrum, which gradually changes to milk over a period of about a fortnight. Compared with the rich, creamy appearance of colostrum and cows' milk, breast milk alone looks thin and 'bluish', but it is always the right quality for your baby, however watery it may appear. The hormones involved in breastfeeding may delay the return of your periods for some months, though ovulation and therefore conception can still occur.

How the baby gets the milk

The baby gets milk by pressing with his gums on milk sacs which lie beneath the areola. The warmth of his mouth relaxes the nipple and milk flows out. As he sucks, hormones are released, causing more milk to flow into his mouth from deeper inside the breast, and often to drip from the other breast. At the same time you may notice a tingling sensation in the nipple and a feeling of fullness in the breast. This sensation is known as the 'let-down reflex'. Not only does it control the milk flow, it is also the signal for more milk to be made. A first-time mother may not be aware of the let-down reflex at first, but if you have had a baby before you may recognize the sensation within a few days of starting to breastfeed.

Once the let-down reflex has been established it can be set off by the baby taking the breast, and also by hearing him cry or thinking of something connected with him or with feeding. Similarly it can be held back if you are tired, anxious, or in pain, or if the baby does not take the whole nipple and areola into his mouth. When the reflex is working efficiently, the amount of milk is nearly always determined by the demands of the baby. *The more often he sucks, the more milk is made.*

Antenatal advice about breastfeeding

Almost all women are physically able to feed their babies, but many do not do so. Some women are advised not to because of ill-health, and a few find breastfeeding so physically distasteful that they will not do it. Some women have inverted nipples so that the baby has difficulty grasping them in his mouth, but this problem can often be corrected by antenatal treatment. There remain the thousands of women who want to feed their babies, and who try to do so, but who become involved in so many avoidable major and minor crises that they abandon the struggle, often before the baby is a month old. This is very sad. It is true that artificial feeding is usually satisfactory and that most babies thrive on modified cows' milk, but breastfeeding is better.

Antenatal preparation

Well-fitting bra During pregnancy you will need one or even two changes to a larger bra size. Don't buy a bra without first trying it on. It should fit well, supporting the breasts underneath and at the sides, without pressing on the nipple. The straps should be wide and firm, to support the extra weight without cutting into your shoulders, and adjustable at the front. Most women find cotton more comfortable than synthetic fabrics. Special maternity bras can be worn during pregnancy as well as during lactation. The Mava Bra, designed and sold by the NCT, is highly recommended and comes in a very large range of cup-sizes and rib-cage fittings. You should wear your maternity bra at night as well as during the day from the seventh month of pregnancy, or earlier if the breasts are enlarged or heavy.

Washing Your regular bath, shower, or daily all-over wash is the only cleansing the nipples require, both now and later. Use soap sparingly as it is a drying agent which could increase the chance of having cracked nipples later. A little pure lanolin, baby oil, or nipple cream gently massaged into the nipples daily will help keep them supple. Avoid using toilet water, which is alcohol-based and could cause dry skin.

Preparing your breasts for feeding Though the days are mercifully gone when women were told to scrub their nipples with nail-brushes 'to toughen them up' it is still necessary to prepare them for the treatment they will undergo during breastfeeding. Pull out each nipple gently and roll it between your thumb and forefinger, once or twice a day, being sure not to cause pain. Stimulation of the nipples while making love has the same helpful effect as well as being pleasurable.

Some women do not like to handle their breasts during pregnancy. Don't worry if you, too, feel that it is distasteful. The natural oils produced by the skin will lubricate your nipples, as long as you do not use soap or any other drying agents on them.

Expressing colostrum Colostrum, the fluid secreted before the milk comes in, may form crusts on the nipples during pregnancy which should be washed off gently. It can be useful to know how to express during late pregnancy in case you need to do it after your baby is born. If you wish to do this, only do it for a minute or two on each side since there may be very little fluid at this stage, especially in a first pregnancy.

One of the easiest times to learn how to express is in the bath. Lean forward and let your breasts hang down. Support one breast in one hand and, with the other hand, place the tips of the thumb and forefinger (or middle finger) on opposite sides of the areola, just on the outer edge. Feeling gently, you will find small, firm 'lumps' – the milk reservoirs where the colostrum, and later the milk collects. Pressing inwards, squeeze the reservoirs gently between your finger and thumb, and beads of colostrum will appear on the nipple. Remember this is something you have to learn to do: it may not work the first time you try. The emphasis is on gentleness: if it hurts, you are not doing

Expressing colostrum

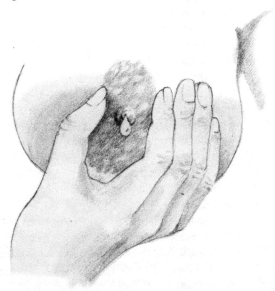

it properly. Don't worry if you cannot express at this stage; it won't affect your ability to breastfeed.

Flat or inverted nipples   Your midwife or doctor should have examined your nipples to make sure that they are protractile. They should stand out when they are gently squeezed, when you are cold, and when you are sexually aroused. If you find difficulty in pulling them out they may be flat or inverted, and it is wise to ask your doctor or midwife about this. They may advise you to wear Woolwich Shells: small glass or plastic cups which fit over the nipple and draw it out by pressing gently on the areola. Use them according to the instructions provided with the shells, which can be obtained from good chemists, ordered from John Bell and Croyden, Wigmore Street, London WC1, or prescribed by your doctor.

Points to remember   Before you give birth, be sure to tell whoever is going to conduct your confinement that you want to breastfeed. If you are going to a hospital or nursing home, this information will be written on your case notes at the antenatal clinic.

At the birth

If you are given the baby to hold before the placenta comes away, or soon after, you will be able to put him to the breast immediately. Hold him close while you support the breast with your hand. He will turn his head and you can guide the nipple into his mouth.

Suckling immediately after birth helps the uterus to contract, and so expel the placenta naturally and more quickly.

The sucking reflex is at its strongest directly after birth. With every hour that suckling is delayed, the reflex weakens so that the baby progressively knows less and less how to respond when put to his mother's breasts. If it is delayed until the breasts are full and hard, suckling is made more difficult for him and more uncomfortable for the mother, who may need patience and perseverance. The baby is also missing the very valuable colostrum which is the link between placental feeding and the new food – breast milk – that will be nourishing him shortly.

The first suckling may only be for a minute or two each side. There is only a little colostrum in the breasts, but there is enough to satisfy the baby and establish the sucking reflex. He then knows what he has to do when he is put to the breasts a little later.

Demand feeding If you are in a hospital which carries out demand feeding, or allows a baby to be beside his mother's bed, you will be able to feed him when he wakes and cries. If the babies are put in a nursery, ask if yours may be brought to you for feeding when he cries and not be given a bottle feed of any sort between breastfeeds. Extra milk will spoil his appetite and he will not suck strongly at the breasts, which will then miss the necessary stimulation to keep up the supply of milk.

Make sure all the staff know that you want your baby brought to you for feeding every time he is hungry. If possible talk, or else write, to the Sister of the postnatal ward about this before your baby is born. If she agrees and thinks it would be helpful, you can have the following notice ready to give her after he is born – to be pinned to the cot:

BABY .... **ENTIRELY BREASTFED PLEASE**
(Your surname)

Mother willing to feed at any time, day or night.

Once your milk has come in, if the staff think (because of his weight) that he is not having sufficient, suggest that they let him feed more frequently. This is much better than giving an extra feed in a bottle, *as more frequent suckling increases the supply*. In that way, your supply will build up to meet his need and you will be able to return to less frequent feeding.

For expectant fathers

Pregnancy is a time when there are significant developments in every marriage which can put stress on even the happiest relationships. It is as though the invisible bonds which join a loving couple must be untied and reassembled to make that couple into a family. During pregnancy, the expectant mother usually gets a lot of support from her family and friends, from her doctor, the hospital, and her antenatal class, but her husband's need for support during this maturing process is not usually recognized.

This book, and this chapter, are written to help you understand your feelings, and your wife's, during her pregnancy.

Pregnancy

Many couples are torn between wanting to start a family and facing a change in their lifestyle: your wife may have to give up her job and you will have to face much greater financial responsibility. Your wife may also miss her working friends and, while she is waiting for the baby to be born, find cleaning and cooking a poor substitute for the stimulus of a job outside the home.

A first pregnancy is a challenge to the couple's ability, not only to make adjustments to their way of life, but also to cope with major changes in the mother's body. During the first three months she will not look pregnant but will be acutely aware of her pregnancy from the moment it has been diagnosed. She may be sick or sleepy – or on the other hand, she may hardly have any physical symptoms. In this case she will resent being mollycoddled but should still be encouraged to rest more than usual. As the baby grows and develops, chemical changes take place stimulated by the glands which also play a part in controlling the emotions. During pregnancy most women are, therefore, much more emotionally on edge than usual. You will probably find the middle three months are a more stable period.

Try to keep up her morale during the last few weeks by finding interesting things to do together – especially if she passes her estimated date of delivery. To her, each 'extra' day will seem like an age, so be patient and understanding if she is grumpy and frustrated. She may need reassurance that you still find her attractive in spite of the bulk of her body.

Before your wife goes for her regular antenatal visits, talk things over so that if either of you has any queries she can make a note and ask them during her examination. You may like to accompany her – antenatal clinics increasingly welcome the husband's interest. Remind her to carry out any particular advice she has been given and encourage her to keep to a healthy diet (see p. 36).

She will probably be invited to go to preparation classes at her hospital or local clinic, and may also wish to attend NCT classes. Encourage her to go and then to tell you the things she has learned. A woman can give birth without knowing anything about the process, but it can be very frightening and unpleasant. A good course of antenatal preparation will help her to train her mind and her body to cope with the experiences of pregnancy and labour. Attend classes with her if you can: some antenatal teachers teach couples, while others include a father's evening in the course. You will learn many interesting facts to refute the horror stories with which expectant parents are bombarded, plus hints on recognizing the onset of labour and lots of suggestions for making things easier for both of you.

Discuss beforehand whether you wish to be together during labour, and find out what steps you should take to make this possible. Slides or a film of a birth may clarify your ideas, but not everyone wants to see someone else's baby delivered before they see their own – the emotional commitment is just not comparable. Many men have a distorted idea of the amount of blood and suffering in labour and feel they would hate to witness it. They do not realize how involved they will feel inside the room, doing something helpful, rather than pacing the corridor outside. Many couples feel that sharing this experience of birth has given a deeper meaning to their relationship and to their feelings for the child. The vast majority of husbands rate it one of the most important experiences of their lives. If you do wish to be together, be sure to discuss the idea with your doctor and midwife and seek their permission before the onset of labour. A well-prepared father can be of assistance to the nursing staff as well as to the mother.

Long before the expected date of delivery discuss how your child will be fed. More and more women are wishing to feed their babies naturally, and reading informed facts about breast-feeding (p. 140) will help give you both confidence. A woman who cannot breastfeed her baby, for physical or emotional reasons, needs your support too. If your wife is not sure how to feed the baby, encourage her to breastfeed, at least for the first few days, when the fluid in her breasts (colostrum) is especially valuable for your baby's health and digestion.

Prelude to labour

It is wise to have everything ready for the baby three weeks before the due date. Your wife will feel happier if she has a telephone number where she can reach you during the day or, if this is not possible, the number of a friend who is willing to sit with her during early labour. Pin a list of the telephone numbers of midwives, doctors, hospital, and ambulance by your telephone. If you have no telephone, keep some coins of the right size for your local call-box in a convenient place. If you plan to drive your wife to the hospital, check petrol and tyres regularly. Keep a couple of cushions and a rug in the car and make sure you are familiar with the best routes to the admission block, both by night and during rush hours.

If the baby is to be born at home, check your fuel supply and make sure that you have fuse-wire and an alternative source of heat for the bedroom available in winter. Your wife may need some extra pillows and the midwife might find a bedside lamp or powerful torch useful.

The onset of labour

You will have read about the three common signs that labour is beginning: regular contractions felt as menstrual cramp, backache, or wind; the 'show' or blood-streaked plug of jelly from the cervix (which may appear some days before labour is established), and the gushing or breaking of the waters. Many women, however, do not have these definite signs and it is difficult to decide when the vague intermittent sensations, which the early contractions of the uterus give rise to, are the 'real thing'. Wait until the contractions become longer, stronger, and at shorter intervals, before notifying the hospital or sending for the midwife. If the confinement is to be at home, make sure that your house is warm and well-lit and that light refreshments are available. If you are going into hospital to stay with your wife, you may need warm clothing for a chilly night vigil but later be glad to strip down to a cotton shirt if you are going into the delivery room. You may like to prepare and take with you a bag containing:

Frozen picnic freezing bag to put against you wife's back if she has backache.

Small natural sponge to moisten her mouth.

Lipsalve or vaseline to prevent her lips becoming chapped.

Jigsaws, books, playing cards, etc., in case it is a long-drawn-out labour with long gaps between contractions.

A vacuum flask of cracked ice for her to suck during labour (to make it more refreshing, the ice could be made from water containing some fresh fruit juice).

Refreshments – drinks, sandwiches, etc., for you, with enough left for her to have after the birth if she has just missed a hospital mealtime.

Change for the hospital telephone box.

(You should keep the bag containing these things, since your wife's belongings may be removed for safekeeping.)

Labour

You will find a clear description of the course of labour on pp. 69–91, with suggestions about how both parents can cope with the sequence of events.

As labour advances, a woman's thoughts are focused on what is happening to her body, and she has no time for the niceties of behaviour. Her emotions are near the surface and may easily spill over into laughter or tears, particularly at the moment of birth. She may swear or snap at you during the transition phase. Take it all in good part and adapt to meet her needs; you are in a better position than anyone else to do this. In a hospital, nurses have other patients and other duties to attend to, you have only your wife. If you are quiet and obviously competent, they will welcome your presence. Stand up for your wife's wishes, but do not be aggressive: this will only antagonize the staff. If you want something, get it by charm.

When you are present at the delivery, don't be surprised if you, too, don't know whether to laugh or to cry. It is an unforgettable experience to see your newborn child come into the world. New babies may be deep pink or even purple, be wrinkled like old men, show traces of blood or the white cream which covered them while they were in the uterus, and their heads can be a peculiar shape with a bump at the back. The genitals of a newborn baby often seem unexpectedly large, If you have never seen a very young child, make a point of looking at some colour photographs of new babies. They do not look at all like the chubby, smiling cherubs in glossy advertisements.

Personal experience

A father wrote this shortly after the birth of his child:

'A postcript for future fathers

Regardless of where the baby is being born, at home or hospital, be prepared to leave your sense of embarrassment somewhere else – you will soon realize that what is happening to your wife is the most real thing she has ever experienced.

She will do things which, under normal circumstances would be ludicrous, she will groan and moan softly or loudly, she may become totally uninterested in you, she will ask you questions you have no answers for ("How much longer?") . . . so, since she is putting her whole self into her labour it will help her and you if you become as totally involved as possible. You can help her greatly by answering questions the nurses ask and by making the decisions – she is in no state to think about anything but what is happening to her body. And above all, be positive. Never cast even the shadow of a doubt into her mind. Always tell her that she is doing well, because no matter what she is doing she is doing the best she can. Do not judge her – help her, give her some of your energy.

The amount of togetherness you discover during the birth of your child will remain with you and grow for the rest of your lives.'

LABOUR & BIRTH

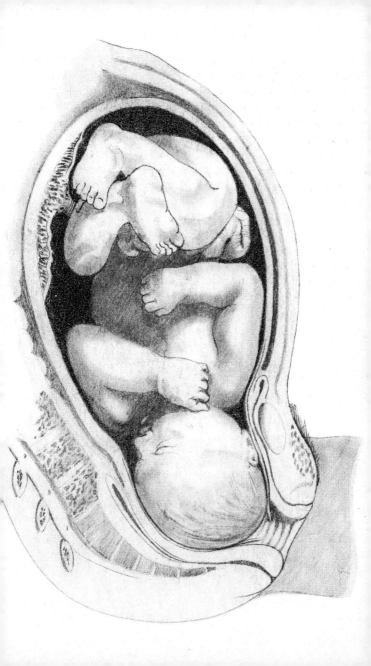

Introduction

Having a baby is hard physical work and emotionally demanding. It is possible to do it without any knowledge or training but, unless you are very lucky, the experience may be traumatic if you undergo it with no idea how to help yourself. It is like being thrown in the deep end of a swimming pool and being expected to struggle to the side. National Childbirth Trust antenatal preparation can never guarantee you an easy birth, but it does offer confidence-giving knowledge, practical information, a range of useful suggestions for coping with labour, and a chance to talk freely about your expectations and worries. Only a tiny minority of women experience no discomfort at all in labour, but many feel that actively working with their own bodies during this unique experience gives them lasting satisfaction and pride. Labour is not a test, however, to be 'passed' or 'failed' according to the degree of pain, and NCT antenatal classes never aim to make you feel guilty if you have to accept analgesic drugs or have complications which entail the use of the full battery of modern life-saving techniques. Indeed, you are taught at classes how best to co-operate with these procedures.

Your husband can learn how to be an active and useful helper during your labour, so that you may feel that you have lived through the experience together and have made your relationship richer and deeper.

Though many women prefer to have their babies in hospital, you may wish to have your baby at home. For low-risk cases, this is an option to consider, provided your home conditions are suitable and there is a maternity hospital within easy reach.

Sometimes, of course, complications arise in giving birth. Some babies have to be born by Caesarean section and, if this happens, you will have to cope with post-operative pain and other discomforts as well as the usual joys and stresses of early motherhood. Many women nowadays have to cope with the pain caused by stitches in the perineum after the birth outlet has been enlarged by an incision during delivery: this is especially true for a woman having her first baby or a forceps delivery.

Medical research is now showing what ordinary mothers could have testified for generations: that uninterrupted early contact between you and your newborn baby is important for you both.

The anatomy and physiology of labour

Labour is the process of childbirth which occurs at the end of pregnancy, usually about 40 weeks from the date of your last period. Three stages of labour can be identified, each of which has a specific function. The first stage pulls up and opens the neck of the uterus, called the cervix. The second stage is the journey of your baby along the birth canal, from the uterus to the outside world. The third stage involves the delivery of the afterbirth, or placenta, which completes the process.

The first stage

This is usually the longest part of labour, and with a first baby averages about ten hours. Subsequent babies average six to eight hours, but as labours vary considerably these times can only be a guide to you.

In order to pull up and open the cervix, the muscular uterus has to contract, producing contractions also known as 'labour pains'. In the last weeks of pregnancy, the uterus becomes thicker towards the top and thinner at the bottom. You may feel it tighten periodically at this time, as it makes preparatory contractions. The tubular cervix is taken up by the uterus, until it is only an opening at the lower end. The plug of mucus, the 'show', which has sealed the cervix during pregnancy, then becomes loosened and falls out.

During labour the muscle fibres of your uterus contract, becoming shorter and fatter. However, when they relax between contractions they do not resume their original size but remain slightly smaller, so that the uterus gradually gets smaller with each contraction. Early contractions are often felt as low, intermittent backache, or period-type pain. Later, the feeling centres at the top of your 'bump', and more greatly resembles cramp. Contractions are also visible: the 'bump' becomes hard and appears to bulge forward. If you place your hand lightly upon it, you will feel this sensation heralding a contraction. How painful these contractions are is very subjective, but knowledge of their function, combined with conscious relaxation, can help you considerably. Every labour is individual, and it is never wise to prejudge the experience by the experiences of others.

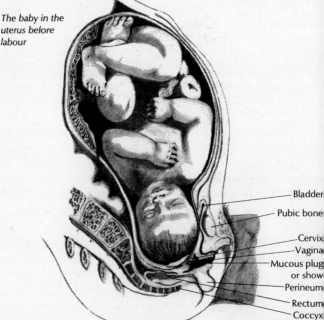

The baby in the uterus before labour

Bladder

Pubic bone

Cervix

Vagina

Mucous plug or show

Perineum

Rectum

Coccyx

The uterus continues to contract, each time opening the cervix wider. The contractions become more frequent, then more intense. At the height of labour, they may come every five minutes, lasting about two minutes, and followed by about three minutes' interval, that is, twelve per hour, with rest for thirty-six of the sixty minutes. This is a typical sequence, but the times may vary in each case.

As far as the baby is concerned, all this has the effect of living in a gradually deflating balloon, slowly but surely being directed towards the opening.

The bag of fluid protecting the baby helps to open the cervix by exerting firm, even pressure on it. At some point the pressure on the membraneous bag will become too great, and it will rupture, the warm fluid gushing or leaking forth, depending on

The waters about to break (the baby's head now rests inside the cervix)

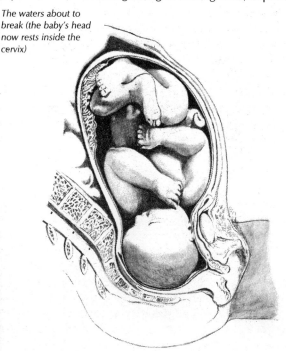

how fully the baby's head is plugging the cervix. This process may be helped if the mother remains upright for as long as possible during labour.

Guides to the first stage

These symptoms may happen in any order or combination:

Show   This is clear, white, pink, or brown mucus, sometimes streaked with blood, and about the size of a thimble. It is often flushed away when passing urine, and may not even be noticed. Alone, it is not an urgent sign and, unless accompanied by bright red bleeding, all that is necessary is to note when it happened and to check that all is prepared.

Contractions   Regular contractions of the uterus, continued over some time, are a definite sign of labour. At first they may only be weak and irregular, often stopping and restarting after a few hours. Unless you are specifically advised to the contrary, continue your usual activities steadily until the contractions are lasting for about three-quarters of a minute each, or are causing concern, at which time you should contact the midwife, and go to the place where your baby is to be born.

Waters breaking/ruptured membranes   This may happen as a first indication of labour, or it may not happen until later. Once the amniotic sac has ruptured and the cervix is dilated, there is a direct passage into the world for the baby and the midwife should be contacted without delay.

Transition to the second stage

There may be a transition phase at the end of the first stage of labour and before the second stage begins, when there is a change from contractions which open the cervix to those which push out the baby. This phase is often signalled by contractions which do not follow a pattern and which have increased intensity. It may be accompanied by nausea, vomiting, mental confusion, and a premature urge to bear down. The transition phase may last for one contraction or perhaps up to an hour, but it is not noticed in every labour.

The second stage

Once established, the second stage is one in which the labour-ing woman can work with her body, responding to the usually strong urge to bear down with each contraction. Many women find this stage both enjoyable and painless. There is no longer any resistance from the cervix, and each contraction pushes the baby a fraction of the four inches along the birth canal. It may take one to two hours for a first baby, or perhaps only one or two contractions with subsequent ones. The birth canal is curved and good positioning is important to bring gravity to bear. If you are flat on your back, the baby will have to travel uphill for part of his journey. If you sit up, well-supported, you can more easily help to push the baby towards birth.

The baby in the birth canal

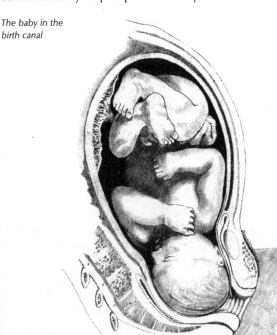

As the baby is manoeuvred along with each push, the accordion-like folds of the vagina open out in front of his head, tucking themselves back into position as he passes on his way. Eventually he reaches the end of the birth canal and, with chin on chest, stretches the vaginal opening with the back of his head, emerging as if through the neck of a tight pullover. At this point you are asked not to bear down, so that the baby is born without undue haste and avoiding possible damage to your perineal skin. Once his head is born, his shoulders twist round in the birth canal and his head turns upwards. The midwife checks that the umbilical cord is not hindering progress. One after the other his shoulders emerge, and his body slithers

The baby's head about to be born

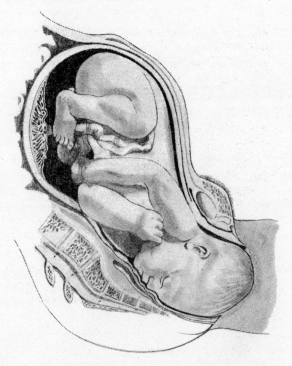

out. Thus he changes from expected baby to newborn, some-times protesting loudly, sometimes just viewing the world with a quizzical air.

His cord is clamped and separated, and he passes into the welcome of your arms.

The third stage

The final stage of labour is the delivery of the placenta. As the baby is being born, an injection is usually given to hasten the third stage, which may only take ten to fifteen minutes to complete. (This injection is a hormone, usually ergometrine and oxytocin, which helps the uterus to contract strongly.) As

The birth of the head (the head rotates sideways as it emerges)

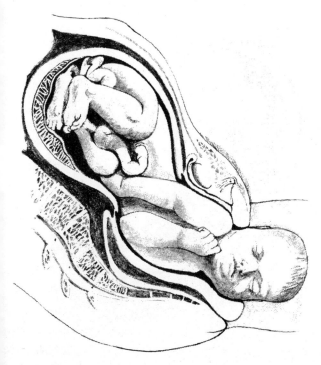

your uterus has decreased in volume, the area to which the placenta has clung has also decreased. When the baby no longer distends the uterus, it becomes much smaller, and the placenta is pushed off completely. The midwife notes external signs of this, and asks you to bear down with the next contraction, sometimes pulling gently on the cord, until the placenta arrives complete.

The contractions become irregular and subside. Although the placental site will continue to leak for several days, like menstruation, the uterus will have contracted sufficiently to prevent any excessive bleeding. If the baby sucks at the breast immediately after birth, it helps the uterus to contract.

The delivery of the placenta

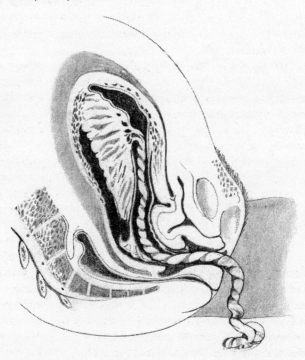

Breathing patterns

The instinctive reaction in time of stress is to tense up and hold your breath. This is helpful for a threatened animal who has to choose between fight or flight, but is generally unhelpful for human beings in stress situations, and it is particularly unhelpful in labour.

The labouring woman cannot escape the powerful sensations within her body as her uterus begins its tremendous task of opening up and pushing her baby into the world. Fighting these sensations is distressing and tiring. Concentrating on relaxing and breathing helps the woman to accept her contractions and the pattern of her labour.

There are many ways of teaching breathing for labour, but the basic principles of varying the rhythm and depth to provide enough oxygen and make the mother comfortable and relaxed are the same.

The patterns are not difficult or tiring, they simply make use of normal breathing rhythms and depths. When you use a lot of energy, you breathe deeply because extra oxygen is needed to enable your muscles to work, and you breathe out extra carbon dioxide as the waste product of your activity. For moderate activity you breathe less deeply, using approximately the upper two-thirds of the lungs to supply fresh air for your needs and to get rid of stale air. The shallowest breathing pattern is used when you are resting, relaxed, and perhaps dropping off to sleep, then you use only the top of the lungs and there is a gentle rise and fall at the top of the chest.

Breathing is controlled by the diaphragm, which is a big muscle, shaped like an upside-down soup plate, stretching right across the body below the ribs. This flattens downwards as breath is taken in and arches upwards and away from the stomach as air is breathed out. In labour, when the abdomen is full of the hard contracting muscle of the uterus, it can become uncomfortable to breathe deeply. So, although some women find that slow deep breathing is all they need in the first stage of labour, most find that as the contractions become stronger, breathing is easier if it is lightened and made a little faster so that the diaphragm does not press on the uterus. Even shallower breathing can be used at the peak of strong contractions, and if this is not effective it is useful to concentrate on counting or on mouthing the words of a song, and to let the breathing take care of itself. Towards the end of the first stage, when there may be a need to control the urge to push, a breathing rhythm incorporating crisp blowing can be used. In the second stage the woman can join in with her uterus to push her baby out, and this is easier if she has learnt how to use her breath effectively. At the third stage she uses the diaphragm which she has been relaxing during early labour.

How to practise breathing patterns

Settle yourself comfortably, propped up and well supported by cushions, as for practising relaxation. Spend a little time relaxing your body and becoming aware of your breathing. Make especially sure that your mouth and jaw are relaxed. Most women find it helpful to learn to concentrate on the 'out' breath. This helps to avoid over-breathing.

Deep breathing (sometimes called easy or complete breathing, or level A)   Sigh out a long, slow breath, feeling your ribs gently squeezing your lungs, like fingers round two sponges, pause, and then gently breathe in to refill your lungs. As your lungs expand you will feel your lower chest swelling and probably your abdomen too! Sigh out again, calmly and peacefully releasing tension as well as air, breathe in easily, sigh out . . . in through your slightly open mouth, and out through your mouth. Do it at a rate and depth which is comfortable for you and spend time getting to know your rhythm. Some people, particularly those practised in yoga, prefer to do this breathing in and out through their noses. See which way works best for you and practise it. By and large, the slower and more relaxed, the better.

When you are happy with that you can move on to:

Shallower breathing (sometimes called middle chest or bellows breathing, or level B)   Next time you sigh out, keep your mouth open and let the air come back into your lungs through your

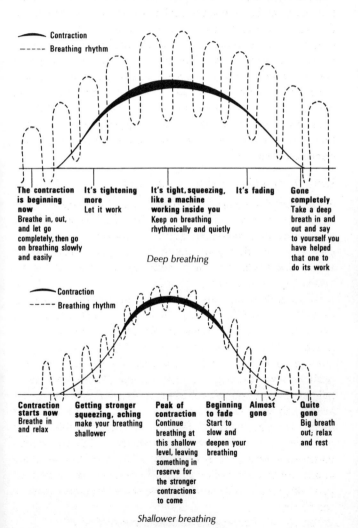

--- Contraction
--- Breathing rhythm

The contraction is beginning now
Breathe in, out, and let go completely, then go on breathing slowly and easily

It's tightening more
Let it work

It's tight, squeezing, like a machine working inside you
Keep on breathing rhythmically and quietly

It's fading

Gone completely
Take a deep breath in and out and say to yourself you have helped that one to do its work

Deep breathing

--- Contraction
--- Breathing rhythm

Contraction starts now
Breathe in and relax

Getting stronger squeezing, aching
make your breathing shallower

Peak of contraction
Continue breathing at this shallow level, leaving something in reserve for the stronger contractions to come

Beginning to fade
Start to slow and deepen your breathing

Almost gone

Quite gone
Big breath out; relax and rest

Shallower breathing

mouth, sigh out again and just let your lungs expand. There is a sideways movement to the ribs, rather like someone opening a pair of bellows and then slowly squeezing them, gently playing with the flames of a fire, in a steady rhythm. The speed is a little quicker than deep breathing but still rather slow.

Then you can try:

Shallow breathing (sometimes called mouth-centred or upper chest breathing, or level C) With your mouth and tongue really soft and relaxed, make a little 'haa' breath out, let a little air in and 'haa' it out again, as though you were playing with the air in your mouth. You are using the top of your lungs. Movement may be felt or seen at the top of the chest. Make sure you are allowing a little air back in to 'haa' out again. Experiment with your rate and depth until you find what is comfortable for you. Some people like a steady 'haaing' rhythm, and others find

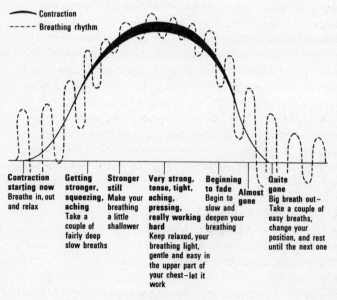

Shallow breathing

easier in threes, 'haa haa haa' – pause – 'haa haa haa' – pause, tc. To reduce the drying effect this shallow breathing has, put ìe tip of your tongue behind your upper teeth.

Now try moving smoothly from the deep breathing through ìe middle breathing to the shallow breathing and back again. ome people envisage lifting their breathing in a rhythm with /aves in the sea, some concentrate on the movements within ìemselves, and some liken it to changing gear in a car.

All this is easier to learn if you have someone to help you. 'ou can actively involve your helper if he or she sits behind you s you either lie well over on your side or sit in front of them, so ìat their hands can rest firmly on your back as you try the ·reathing. Your helper's hands should rest just below your /aist when you are doing the *deep breathing*, in the middle of our back, feeling your ribs for the *shallower breathing*, and ıst below the nape of your neck for the *shallow breathing*. The ıelper will feel a certain amount of movement each time – ìough very slight for the shallow breathing.

ı *distraction* (sometimes called tune tapping, muttering, or ?vel D)   Choose a song or poem with a good beat and mutter : under your breath, concentrating on the activity round your ìouth or on the words, and let your breath come and go as it /ill (you will probably find that you are breathing fairly deeply).)r you can count backwards in the same way and you may ke to add the activity of lightly tapping your fingers in time.

Controlling the urge to push (or transition phase breathing) Jow you can modify the shallow breathing to create a broken ìythm, by adding one or two crisp 'hoo' breaths, like blowing ·ut a match:

ıaa haa hoo, haa haa hoo, haa haa hoo, etc., or

ıaa haa hoo hoo, haa haa hoo hoo, haa haa hoo hoo, etc. ome people find it easier to do a counting rhythm, 1-2 1-2 hoo, -2 1-2 hoo, etc. Choose the one you find most comfortable and ·ractise that.

Beware of *over-breathing or hyperventilating* while you are ·ractising or in labour. This means that you are breathing in too

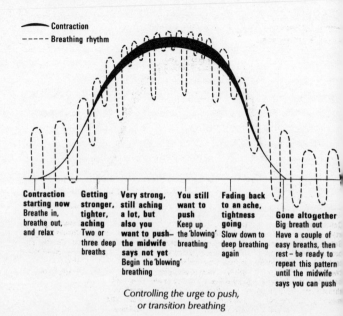

— Contraction					
---- Breathing rhythm					

Contraction starting now
Breathe in, breathe out, and relax

Getting stronger, tighter, aching
Two or three deep breaths

Very strong, still aching a lot, but also you want to push— the midwife says not yet
Begin the 'blowing' breathing

You still want to push
Keep up the 'blowing' breathing

Fading back to an ache, tightness going
Slow down to deep breathing again

Gone altogether
Big breath out
Have a couple of easy breaths, then rest – be ready to repeat this pattern until the midwife says you can push

*Controlling the urge to push,
or transition breathing*

much oxygen and upsetting the oxygen/carbon dioxide balance in your body. You may be aware of dizziness, numbness round your mouth, or tingly fingers. Breathe into your hands cupped over your nose and mouth to counteract this, but also check that your shoulders are really relaxed and that you are breathing gently and concentrating on the 'out' breath.

Breathing for pushing Get into the well-supported position for pushing. Take in one or two easy breaths and let them go, take in another and this time hold it, let your head drop forward so that your chin is resting on your chest and your diaphragm presses down on the baby, relaxing your pelvic floor. You may need two or more breaths during each contraction but remember that it is long sustained pushes that help the birth, so try to keep leaning on the baby even when you are letting the air out and taking another breath in. You may like one or two breaths between pushes. Some women find that they are aware

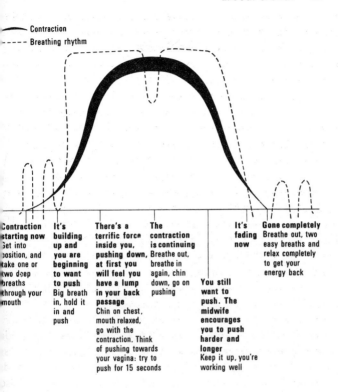

— Contraction

---- Breathing rhythm

Contraction starting now	It's building	There's a terrific force	The contraction		It's fading	Gone completely

Contraction starting now
Get into position, and take one or two deep breaths through your mouth

It's building up and you are beginning to want to push
Big breath in, hold it in and push

There's a terrific force inside you, pushing down, at first you will feel you have a lump in your back passage
Chin on chest, mouth relaxed, go with the contraction. Think of pushing towards your vagina: try to push for 15 seconds

The contraction is continuing, Breathe out, breathe in again, chin down, go on pushing

You still want to push. The midwife encourages you to push harder and longer
Keep it up, you're working well

It's fading now

Gone completely
Breathe out, two easy breaths and relax completely to get your energy back

Breathing for pushing

of the uterus pushing in waves within the contraction and they find alternately holding the breath to push and lightly panting while waiting for the next wave, is most effective for them.

If you have difficulty working out how to push, squat down on the floor and give a cough, you will feel your diaphragm pushing on to the baby and your pelvic floor bulge downwards. Now do that without coughing and sustain it, then you can combine it with the breathing.

Breathing to stop pushing   As the widest part of the baby's head is emerging (the 'crowning') the midwife will probably ask

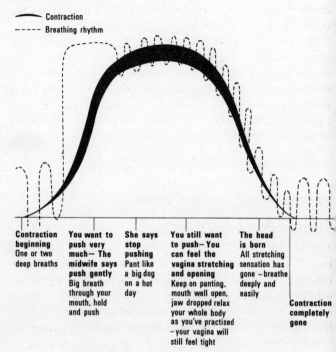

—— Contraction
- - - - Breathing rhythm

Contraction beginning	You want to push very much—	She says stop pushing	You still want to push—	The head is born

Contraction beginning
One or two deep breaths

You want to push very much— The midwife says push gently Big breath through your mouth, hold and push

She says stop pushing Pant like a big dog on a hot day

You still want to push— You can feel the vagina stretching and opening Keep on panting, mouth well open, jaw dropped relax your whole body as you've practised – your vagina will still feel tight

The head is born All stretching sensation has gone – breathe deeply and easily

Contraction completely gone

Breathing to stop pushing (during delivery of the head)

you to stop pushing or to pant. Practise responding to this request immediately, by lifting your chin slightly and panting gently. Be ready to start pushing again as soon as you are told you may.

Using the breathing patterns

Self-help in labour comes from relaxation, breathing and massage. Give yourself and your body time to learn these new skills. Practise them a little *every day* for, say, the last eight weeks of your pregnancy. When labour arrives you may find that your owns skills are all you need to cope with it, but all the extra aids for reducing pain by drugs are still available if and when they are needed and will be even more effective if understood and used to support your own ability to give birth.

These breathing patterns may stand you in good stead in other situations: deep breathing may help you to catnap during the day and get off to sleep between night feeds; shallow breathing may help you when the baby is restless and you feel you are getting tense, and may also help you to keep calm and think straight when everything seems to be going wrong.

A guide to labour for expectant   parents

This is the outline of a normal confinement. Labour is a highly individual affair and no exact pattern can be guaranteed. Do not expect a set series of events but be prepared to accept whatever your particular labour brings. Whatever happens, enjoy as much of it as you can. Particularly, *enjoy knowing what to do to help yourself as much as you are able.* Set yourself no other aims.

In this guide, each phase of labour is set out in distinct parts: 'What is happening', 'Helping yourself', 'Breathing pattern', and 'Husband's help'. This is done for quick and easy reference, and to tie together the subjects we have mentioned separately in previous sections. If you are reading this book early in pregnancy some of the breathing methods may mean little to you. You will learn about them at your antenatal classes.

Prelude to labour

What is happening   You may notice some of the following signs: lightening, when the baby's head drops into the pelvis, two to four weeks before the birth; hardening of your abdomen when the uterus starts frequent 'practice' contractions; increased mucus discharge from the vagina; a weight loss of two to three pounds, three or four days before labour begins;

less activity from the baby; a spurt of energy in you, the mother, one to two days before labour; wind in the bowel, sometimes with slight diarrhoea; pelvic pressure.

Helping yourself   Conserve your energy and simplify the housekeeping. Practise breathing deeply and easily with any contractions you notice, and keep up all practising as advised at your antenatal classes. Have your hospital suitcase packed when you are eight months pregnant; for a home confinement, air the baby clothes, cot blankets and sheets, and have your maternity pack and personal requirements handy in the bedroom. Protect your mattress in case your waters break before labour begins. Don't concentrate too hard on the expected date of confinement, which is after all only a guide. Plan special things for *after* the date – an evening out, or a visit to the hairdresser, or whatever appeals to you and your husband.

Husband's help   Warn the appropriate people at work that you may need some time off or that you will soon be taking part of your holiday. If you have to leave work unexpectedly, make sure someone knows where to contact you if your wife goes into labour. Know all the necessary telephone numbers, and have change ready for the telephone. Know the route to the hospital.

Onset of labour

What is happening   You may notice one, or any combination, of the following: Contractions, felt as backache, period cramp, or similar; the 'show' – a bloodstreaked vaginal discharge; breaking of the waters.

Helping yourself   Check the signs, time the contractions, and report to the midwife or hospital as advised. If the show is very heavy, report it at once. If the waters break, with or without contractions, report this too. In the daytime, continue light activity; at night, rest or, if you feel very excited, get up and make a hot drink, and take a hot water bottle back to bed or lie on a sofa or in an armchair with your feet up. Make sure your hospital case is ready, if you need one.

Husband's help   Check your final preparations (lists may help), and maintain a calm and unhurried atmosphere. Suggest activities of a light nature to avoid a boring wait.

Early first stage

What is happening   The cervix is being drawn up and dilatation is beginning.

Helping yourself   If labour starts slowly, enjoy normal meals, but when contractions are lasting a minute or longer do not eat anything, have only sips of water. If you are in bed, find a good position for relaxation, preferably as upright as possible or on your side, and rearrange your pillows. If it is daytime, rest for each contraction by standing or sitting limply. Continue your household activities gently, or read, watch television, or play with your other children. Concentrating on slow rhythmic breathing often helps.

Breathing pattern   Start slow rhythmic breathing.

Husband's help   At this stage your wife is likely to remain cheerful and to enjoy talking between contractions. Have a meal before leaving for the hospital and take sandwiches with you. Wear cool clothes, not a nylon shirt which will become uncomfortably clammy in the heat of a delivery room.

As the first stage progresses . . .

What is happening   The contractions become stronger and you feel the need to do more about them. They may come more frequently, lasting approximately a minute to a minute and a half. Dilatation continues and the contractions become closer and stronger. The midwife will ask questions about your progress so far, listen to the baby's heart, examine you, and give you a shave and an enema or suppository.

Helping yourself   Go to hospital or, for a home confinement, go to your bedroom and undress. Relax during the journey to the hospital. During the midwife's examination, or while you have an enema, you may have a contraction. If so, ask her to pause until the contraction has gone. Lie or sit in any relaxed

and comfortable position with good back support and turn to
your side if you need back-rubbing. Empty your bladder every
hour or two during the first stage.

Breathing pattern   Slow breathing, becoming shallower as the
contraction gets stronger and deeper as the contraction fades
away.

Husband's help   On arrival at the hospital, help to answer the
staff's questions, and rejoin your wife after she has had her
enema and bath. Encourage her relaxation and breathing,
suggest good positions, and help with massage. She may like
regular feather-light stroking on her tummy, firmer stroking on
the outer or inner thighs, or firm massage on her back (taking
care with this one not to *rub* the skin, but move it over the bones
in a circular motion). Hand lotion on your hands and her skin
makes all these more effective. Explain about breathing control
if your wife cannot answer a question from the staff while she is
coping with a contraction. At this point your wife will be taking
her labour very seriously and may not wish to talk between
contractions.

Late first stage

What is happening   Dilatation continues and the contractions are markedly closer, stronger, and longer. The waters
break now or later, if they have not broken at the start of your
labour.

Helping yourself   Change positions occasionally to find the
most comfortable one, preferably sitting up or half-sitting, half-
lying on your side. Relax during each contraction and let it work.
At the height of the contraction, breathe regularly but more
shallowly or, if necessary, do light, fast breathing. You may be
offered an injection 'to help with relaxation'. If possible discuss
this tactfully before labour; if you are coping easily you can ask
if the injection can be delayed a little. If at any stage you feel
dizzy or have tingling in your fingers or around the mouth,
breathe into cupped hands for a few minutes, then make your
breathing more gentle.

Breathing pattern Establish harmony with the contractions, being prepared to alter your breathing patterns when necessary.

Husband's help Help and encourage your wife's relaxation and breathing. She may prefer you not to talk much or to distract her now, but do explain anything bewildering. Encourage your wife to concentrate. Watch her hands, face, and shoulders, and see that they are relaxed. Continue massage if she likes it. Sips of water and cool sponging of the face will help to keep her alert and coping.

Transition from first to second stage

What is happening Some long, strong, irregular contractions may occur close together, giving you a muddled feeling or an urge to bear down before dilatation is completed. There may also be trembling, cramp in the legs, shivering, sickness, or hiccups. You may feel irritable, angry with everyone, weepy, too hot or too cold: this is all quite normal and a signal that the end of the first stage is approaching and that the birth is likely to happen soon. You may be moved to the delivery room now.

Helping yourself You may be more comfortable sitting up with your legs flopped apart, with or without pillows under your knees, and this will hasten the dilatation of the cervix. Continue with your relaxation, and do not push until the midwife gives permission.

Breathing pattern Concentrate on breathing at the shallow level, responding by blowing out breath whenever the urge to push comes. Soon you will be able to push. Pant, or use controlled blowing breathing, while moving to the delivery room. Instead of the blowing breathing you may prefer to use inhalation analgesia ('gas and oxygen'), with deep breathing through the mouth.

Husband's help Arrange extra pillows to prop up your wife. Remind her that the phase is temporary and heralds the most exciting stage of labour; tell her that when she is allowed to push everything will be much more pleasant. Accept and understand her tears or temper. Do the shallow breathing, blowing out with her when she feels the urge to push, and remind her that this blowing-out breathing can be very definite and purposeful. Your wife may feel out of control of the situation and will look to her attendants for support and guidance during this phase. She will not want to be left alone, and your presence will be especially valuable. Remember to keep yourself relaxed too!

Second stage

What is happening   Your baby is gradually moving down the birth canal; soon his head will be visible. You will probably be able to feel this, and have a strong 'urge to push', although some women do not. The pressure of the baby's head against your rectum may make you feel as if you want to move your bowels, and you may experience a great sense of bulging and stretching. At the crowning of the baby's head there may be a slight burning sensation for a few seconds, or a feeling of numbness as the vaginal opening is stretched tightly. Then as the baby is born you may feel his head sliding out of the vaginal passage, followed by his shoulders and body in the next several contractions. At this stage the midwife will probably give you an injection to help the placenta to separate. She may suck out the baby's mouth to clear the breathing passages.

Helping yourself   Your position is important. Sit up, then rock yourself back, so that the lower part of your back is fairly flat against the bed but your upper back and shoulders are propped up. If there aren't many pillows use them to support your back firmly, rather than your shoulders, which can be supported by your husband or a helper. With your feet hip width apart, bend your knees up and let them flop apart so that your feet are resting on the bed on their outer edges: any pressure on the soles of the feet tightens the pelvic floor muscles and thus makes it more difficult for the baby to get out. You can lightly hold your knees while you push or just let your arms flop at your sides. The midwife will guide you and your uterus will probably dictate the amount of pushing required. Join in, remembering that you are pushing down on your baby and relaxing everything else, especially your pelvic floor. Keep your eyes open and remain alert during the contractions, but rest completely between them. Greet your baby as he is born and touch him as soon as you can.

Breathing pattern　　Hold your breath and push as the contraction demands; pant when the midwife asks you to.

Husband's help　　Give your wife firm encouragement. Rearrange the pillows for a comfortable pushing position, or support your wife with your arm around her shoulders, and remind her to push with her head dropped forward and her mouth soft and relaxed. Help her with relaxation between contractions. Above all, follow the wishes of the doctor or midwife. Welcome the baby, with your wife, when he is born.

Third stage

What is happening　　Less intense contractions occur now and the delivery of the placenta takes place within about 20 minutes. If an injection has been given, the placenta may come away much more quickly. You will be tidied and freshened up.

Helping yourself　　Push to deliver the placenta when the midwife directs you to. Lie back and enjoy your baby! Let him suckle if this is possible.

Afterwards

What is happening　　'After-pains' are felt during the next few days which pull the uterus back into its former shape and almost its former size.

Helping yourself　　Welcome these contractions and if necessary breathe your way over them.

The choice of birth at home

The NCT believes that women should be able to make an informed choice about where they have their babies, and that birth can be an enriching and happy experience either in hospital or at home.

In 1959 the Cranbrook Committee recommended that home confinements should be 30 per cent of the total, but by 1970 only 13 per cent of births in the United Kingdom took place at home, partly because of extra maternity provisions made to cope with what had been a rapidly expanding birth-rate a decade before. Now the birth-rate has declined dramatically, but the hospital beds remain and there is pressure to fill them lest they become uneconomic.

It is fair to say that there are good reasons for having a baby in hospital, as well as good reasons for maintaining a domiciliary service: the high quality for which British midwifery has been justly acclaimed for many years.

Hospital care

There are two different kinds of hospital maternity care: GP units, including cottage hospitals and GP beds attached to or in consultant units, and consultant hospitals, which may have some GP beds in them, and where any mother who is ill or whose baby is at risk would be well advised to go.

Isolated GP units have a safety record slightly below that of home births, but many women like them because they provide a homely atmosphere with a familiar doctor and midwife. If complications occur, the mother has to be moved to a consultant hospital, which should have a special care baby unit attached. If your doctor has already suggested a GP unit confinement, you can infer that you are 'low risk' and that it is safe to have your baby at home.

Good reasons for having a hospital birth

Toxaemia of pregnancy (pre-eclampsia).
A breech presentation   For a home delivery to be relatively safe, the baby should be in a position with its head down before labour starts. With breech presentations the baby's bottom appears first, and the risks involved in delivery are greater.

A previous complicated birth   Sometimes the complications experienced at one delivery will not necessarily be a reason for expecting problems next time. But a Caesarean section or a lot of bleeding after the previous birth are, for instance, reasons for having a subsequent hospital birth.

A premature birth   This is one more than three weeks early, when the baby is likely to be small, and when an incubator and paediatric care should be available. For this reason it is wiser to have twins in hospital, as twins often come early.

Placenta praevia   This is when the placenta is lying in the lower part of the uterus.

The statistics of perinatal mortality

Your doctor will be thinking in terms of perinatal mortality statistics, which indicate stillbirths and all babies who die in the first week of life. In the last year for which detailed study has been done (1970) it was 23 per 1,000 births in England and Wales.

Statistically the risks are greater when: the mother is unsupported (37 per 1,000 – almost twice that of married women); she is over 35 years old (36 per 1,000 compared with 18–19 per 1,000 if she is between 20 and 30); she is Asian-born (32 per 1,000 compared with 21 per 1,000 for women born in England); she is the wife of an unskilled worker (she is four times more likely to lose her baby than the wife of a professional man – 28 per 1,000 compared with 6 per 1,000); she is less than 5 ft 2 ins (158 cm) tall (25 per 1,000 compared with 17 per 1,000 women over this height); she is having her first baby (23 per 1,000 compared with 16 per 1,000 for a second baby).

Note that even when the perinatal mortality rates are highest, the vast majority of babies are born safely. The safest age at which to have a baby is when the woman is between 20 and 30. For babies born at home the perinatal mortality rate in 1970 was 5 per 1,000, which compares very favourably with the overall rate for the same year of 23 per 1,000. It does not mean that home is safer than hospital, but that women with the most complicated births had their babies in hospital, as they should.

Why home may be a good place

If the pregnancy is straightforward and the labour is likely to be normal, there are some advantages in having a baby at home. These include the practical advantages of avoiding travel to hospital when in labour, and being moved from room to room in hospital; avoiding unnecessary obstetric intervention; avoiding drugs which may adversely affect the baby; being able to keep mobile; and the relative ease in starting breastfeeding in one's own home and outside an institutional environment. There are the emotional benefits of feeling confident and relaxed in a familiar place; having continuity in maternity care; avoiding separation from other children in the family and allowing them to regard birth as a natural part of life; keeping mother and baby close together during the important minutes and hours after delivery; and feeling that you are retaining responsibility for your child's birth, with supportive rather than directive medical help.

The vital factor in preparing for a home confinement is to have the very best antenatal care possible.

How to set about getting a home confinement

The first person to talk to is your doctor, whom you may find understanding and helpful. Many doctors believe, however, that all babies should be born in hospital, and may therefore try to dissuade you from having a home birth – perhaps saying that you are risking the baby's life. (Birth can never be one hundred per cent safe, and of course some babies die wherever they are born. But this is something each couple will want to consider.)

It is a good idea for couples to discuss this together with the doctor, and to write down the advice you are given so that you can think about it coolly afterwards. You do not have to make a snap decision.

The doctor's professional responsibility means that he cannot make firm promises about home confinement early in pregnancy when it cannot yet be known if all will be well in five or six months' time. Most GPs who agree to a home confinement will only do so provided the pregnancy is straightforward. You should be prepared to make it clear to your doctor that you accept and understand this.

The general practitioner obstetrician to whom you go for maternity care need not be your usual GP and you can ask to have maternity care from another GP. Often only one partner in a practice does maternity work anyway. If you are thinking of a home confinement it is worth asking the GP as soon as pregnancy is diagnosed if his or her partner is prepared to do home deliveries provided everything is likely to be straightforward, and if not whether you can have the name of a GP obstetrician who is.

Should your own doctor not know of a GP who does home confinements, you may wish to contact the Area Nursing Officer (at the city or county Health Department) asking for the names of GPs on the obstetric list who sometimes do home confinements. You will probably be put in touch also with the Community Nursing Officer, who supervises the community midwives. Let her know you feel strongly about a home confinement and ask how midwifery cover can be arranged.

If you come to a dead end, write explaining what has happened to your Community Health Council, and ask if they can help. You may like to send copies of your letter to the Area Nursing Officer and to the Family Practitioner Committee, whose address you can get from the Health Department.

According to her conditions of service, established by the Central Midwives' Board, a midwife called when you are in labour at home must attend.

If you already have a GP obstetrician who is opposed to home confinements or if you are attending a consultant unit but want to have a home confinement instead, it is probably best to put your reasons for wanting a home birth in writing to the doctor concerned and to the Area Nursing Officer. Try to be very clear and unemotional about it. It is important that your husband agrees, and a good idea to sign the letter jointly. If your reason for wanting a home confinement is to avoid going to a particular hospital, explain why in detail.

Once a home birth has been agreed, the midwife will look at your home to advise you how to make everything ready. The place should be clean and convenient, with running water, but there is no need to try to reproduce hospital conditions.

As the estimated date approaches, the midwife will leave a sterile maternity pack in your home, and give you any necessary instructions. You will need to provide a bucket and a few bowls and things. There is usually no need to rearrange the bedroom, though it is easier if the bed is at right angles to the wall and can be approached from three sides.

When labour starts   When you feel that your labour is established, contact the midwife. She may ask you to let her know, before she goes out on her rounds in the morning, if you think the baby is likely to be born that day.

Home helps   Social services departments have a statutory duty to provide home helps after home confinements for a period of 14 days – or longer if the GP considers it is necessary. You will have to contribute a certain proportion towards her pay. Your husband may also wish to take a week or more off work.

Sources of further information   You may like to talk to someone who has had a home birth in your area. Other people who may be able to help are: your NCT teacher; The Society to Support Home Confinements, Margaret Whyte, 17 Laburnum Avenue, Durham City; The Patients' Association, Suffolk House, Banbury Road, Oxford; The Association for Improvement in Maternity Services (AIMS), Ms. Christine Beels, 19 Broomfield Crescent, Leeds 6.

Remember . . .   if you plan to have a baby at home it is vitally important to have good antenatal care as well as leading a healthy life during pregnancy. See your doctor regularly and take his advice. Do not take any medicine or tablets without consulting your GP even when you are not absolutely sure you are pregnant (it is in early pregnancy that the worst damage can be done to the foetus). Avoid eating synthetic foods and if you smoke give it up if you possibly can, because nicotine reduces the amount of oxygen that reaches the baby. Go to antenatal classes and learn all you can about helping yourself in labour.

Guide to medical procedures during labour

Admission procedures

Unfortunately a great deal of modern maternity care has become routine. In many hospitals as a matter of course every woman has her pubic and vulval hair shaved off, is given an enema, and is asked to take a bath or shower. None of these procedures is essential, but except in a few places you will be expected to conform. If you wish to avoid any or all of this ritual, you would be well advised to discuss the admission procedure with those who will care for you before your labour begins. You may obtain the assurances you hope for, but if not, at least you will be aware of the attitudes that you will meet and what to expect.

Enemas   It is generally more comfortable in labour and less messy at the birth if your lower bowel is empty. The traditional method is to insert a volume of hot soapy water into the rectum via a rubber tube, but the same emptying of the bowel can be achieved as efficiently and with considerably less indignity and discomfort to the mother with suppositories – small bullet-shaped doses of a substance inserted through the back passage (anus) to cause a motion – or with a tablespoonful of a small volume of liquid enema from a sachet.

Shaving   Shaving your pubic hair off completely is not necessary, but hair around the opening of the vagina should be removed so that it does not become matted with blood, or interfere with stitching. If you wash these parts every day, you can keep them as clean as if you had no hair. However, having said this, you may have an uphill struggle to resist this established procedure. You and your partner may together find the necessary strength to protest.

A bath or shower   This is not essential but you may find it pleasurable. The warmth of the bath water may stimulate your contractions. After the diarrhoea induced by an enema you may feel in need of a cleansing soak in the bath or a refreshing shower.

Management of the first stage of labour

Companionship   Most maternity hospitals now allow fathers to be present throughout labour. The shared experience is invaluable to all three of you: mother, father, and baby. It also gives you continuous support so that you never feel alone. But, in many places, husbands are often asked to leave if any procedure, however minor, is carried out, such as giving an injection or making a vaginal examination. If you want your husband to stay, ask the doctor whether it would be possible. Not infrequently, a nurse or midwife will ask the husband to leave before the doctor comes, on the assumption that the doctor will prefer it that way, whereas the doctor may be happy to allow your husband to stay. Make it clear that the husband wants to stay to help his wife, not to interfere with medical procedures.

Your husband may be asked to put on a hospital gown and to wear a cap and mask.

Food and fluid   It is usual practice in most maternity hospitals to forbid taking food and fluid by mouth during labour, in case you have to have a general anaesthetic at some stage, when you might bring back and inhale what is in your stomach. This is not an unreasonable precaution, especially as you may not feel like eating or drinking very much, and as your stomach empties and digests more slowly in labour. However, your mouth may feel dry and to moisten it is a welcome relief that should not be denied. In some places you will be given a white chalky mixture

(Magnesium trisilicate) to drink every few hours during your labour to make the contents of your stomach less acid, and less likely to damage your lungs should you be given a general anaesthetic and inhale any stomach contents.

Intravenous fluids   Many doctors like women in labour to have a 'drip' of fluid through a needle into a vein (intravenous infusion), because the energy that you use during labour demands a constant supply of fluid.

Vaginal examinations   Progress in labour is judged by noting how often your contractions are coming, and how strong and how long they are. More exactly, progress is assessed by measuring how wide open the cervix is and by noting the way in which the baby's presenting part (the leading bit of the baby, usually the top of the head, or vertex, and rarely the bottom, or breech) descends through the birth canal on internal examination. The opening of the cervix is measured in 1–5 finger-breadths, or 1–10 cm. When the cervix is fully open (dilated to 10 cm) the second stage of labour is said to begin. In some hospitals, it is routine practice to assess dilatation of the cervix by vaginal examination repeated every two to four hours. When the waters break it is usual to make a vaginal examination to make sure that a loop of the baby's umbilical cord has not slipped below the head where it could be compressed. It is also advisable to make sure that the baby is unlikely to arrive within the next three hours by checking the dilatation of the cervix before pain-relieving drugs are given or repeated.

Emptying your bladder   Late in labour, because the bladder is pulled upwards as your cervix opens and the baby's head goes down the birth canal, you may find it difficult to urinate or have no desire to empty your bladder. This is especially true under epidural analgesia. The midwives will keep an eye on this, and if necessary pass a tube (catheter) into your bladder to empty it. Keeping the bladder empty gives more room for the baby's head. '

Analgesia   Most midwives and doctors expect you to require pain relief during labour. If you are admitted at night during early labour, often you will be offered a sleeping tablet. Later on the drug most often used is pethidine in a dose of 100 or 150 mg given by injection. Often pethidine is combined with a tranquillizer or antihistamine, which may help to counteract nausea and vomiting, but which also increases drowsiness and gives a feeling of detachment. Injections of pain-relieving drugs should seldom be repeated more than every four hours. Later on in labour it is wise to find out the progress you have made before having injections, since if the birth of your baby can be expected within three hours the drugs given may delay the onset of his breathing. As birth comes nearer, instead of pain-relieving injections you may breathe a mixture of gas (nitrous oxide) and oxygen, or a mixture of the vapour from a sweet-smelling liquid (trilene) and air, during contractions, to help relieve the pain. This inhaled analgesia should be used right at the beginning of each contraction and only about four or five breaths should be taken so that you are awake to use it at the start of the next contraction.

Many women, particularly those having a second or subsequent baby, find that they can handle their labours without taking any form of drugs, but just using relaxation and breathing techniques. However, labour should never be a mere endurance test, and if you feel in need of extra relief you should not hesitate to ask for it. Since pethidine is a mood-enhancing drug it is best to request it before you become distressed. The time to ask is when you begin to feel that you cannot cope *between contractions*. Pethidine is a poor analgesic, but it can help you to relax and sleep between contractions. Be sure, however, to ask for an examination to find out the dilatation of your cervix, as you may be reaching the end of the first stage in which case the drug would not take effect before you wanted to start to push your baby out in the second stage of labour. Pethidine is known to depress the baby's sucking reflex, so if your baby is sleepy and slow to suck at first, do not worry. The effect of the drug will wear off, and feeding will become much easier.

Epidural analgesia   The   nerves   which   conduct   sensations from the uterus, cervix, and vagina to the brain leave the lower spinal cord, which is surrounded by your backbone (vertebral column). The nerves can be temporarily blocked so that they no longer conduct impulses by exposing them to a solution of local anaesthetic. In epidural anaesthesia this is done by placing a thin plastic tube between two of your lower vertebrae into the spinal canal just outside the spinal cord and near the nerve roots to your lower body and legs. The tube is threaded through a needle, inserted after first numbing your back. Once the plastic tube is in place, the needle is withdrawn and the local anaesthetic solution is injected. You will then feel numb in the lower half of your body and legs. You may still be aware that your uterus is contracting, but you will not feel it as pain. The effect of an epidural varies with the placement of the tube and the dose of anaesthetic used, and usually lasts between one and three hours. When one dose wears off, further doses of the anaesthetic solution can be given through the plastic tube, which is left in place until your baby has been born.

The advantages of epidural analgesia are that you remain fully awake and free from pain without the need for other pain-relieving and sedative drugs. Because epidural analgesia causes a drop in blood pressure, it is useful for women whose blood pressure is high. Epidural analgesia can also be used instead of putting you to sleep with a general anaesthetic to carry out forceps, breech, and twin delivery as well as Caesarean section.

The disadvantages of epidural analgesia are that your movement is restricted, it requires careful supervision, and there is an increased need to use forceps for delivery. Many women with epidurals find it difficult to push their babies out themselves, because they have lost their vaginal sensations. However, you can be helped to push out your baby yourself, if you are guided when to push with your contractions. Epidural analgesia requires special skill and experience, and may not be available at all times, or even at all in some maternity hospitals.

Monitoring the health of your baby   When the waters break, the fluid should be clear, straw-coloured, or milky. Sometimes it contains white greasy flecks – the vernix, which is a protective secretion from the glands of the baby's skin. All this is perfectly normal. If, however, the water that drains out is stained green or dark yellow from the meconium in the baby's bowel, this is a warning that the baby may be short of oxygen and the midwife or doctor will want to make sure that the baby is born soon.

Normally the baby's heart beats at a rate of between 120 and 160 per minute, the actual speed at any moment varying quite considerably between these limits. The heart-rate can be counted by listening to it through a stethoscope or with ultrasound (Sonicaid). During normal labour the baby's heart-rate, your pulse and blood pressure are recorded at first every hour, later every half-hour, and towards the end of labour perhaps after every contraction. In complicated labours warning of danger can be provided if the foetal heart-rate is recorded and observed continuously. This is called monitoring and can be done automatically after picking up the heartbeat from sound or ultrasound waves, or from electrical signals. Usually a receiver for the signals from the baby's heart is strapped to your abdomen, which also records the contractions of your uterus by means of a pressure-sensitive gauge. A cable connects the receiver to a computer which calculates the heart-rate and provides a continuous written record of what is happening. Some obstetricians prefer to record the baby's heart-rate directly by attaching a metal clip to the baby's head through the vagina and cervix after the membranes have ruptured.

Some hospitals follow a policy of monitoring every woman continuously throughout labour. They do this because they believe that it is in the best interests of the baby, but it has the disadvantage that you are unable to get out of bed and it is difficult even in bed to move around freely. It can be argued whether or not real advantage is to be gained by continuous monitoring of every labour, rather than by selecting only those women who have signs of early foetal distress or in whom there is some reason to suspect that the baby may become distressed, for example, women with raised blood pressure, those who have had difficulties in earlier pregnancies, or those who are ten days or more past the expected date of delivery.

Acceleration of labour   Labour lasting more than 24 hours is not generally good, either for you or your baby. If uterine contractions are weak, infrequent and/or irregular, they can be made more effective in dilating the cervix by dripping the hormone oxytocin (Syntocinon) into a vein at a carefully measured rate. Many obstetricians believe that more than 12 hours in labour is undesirable, and will, therefore, accelerate labour sooner than other doctors who are willing for labour to last a little longer. The rate of progress in labour generally speeds up after the membranes rupture. The membranes can be ruptured artificially for this purpose by nicking a hole in them as they bulge through the opening cervix with a pair of forceps passed along the fingers during a vaginal examination.

The second stage of labour

You may feel that the second stage is the really positive part of your labour, when you can work with your body to bring your baby into the world. You may value your husband's support and companionship particularly now and want to share with him the moving experience of the delivery itself.

An episiotomy   This is a cut made in the skin and muscles to enlarge the opening to the vagina so that the baby's head can pass out more easily and/or more quickly. An episiotomy should not usually be made without first numbing the tissues that are to be cut by injecting a local anaesthetic solution. Many obstetricians encourage the almost routine use of episiotomy, especially in women having their first babies, although other obstetricians maintain that this is not necessary. Episiotomies *are* necessary if they are needed to protect you and your baby from injury, for example, if the baby is born too early (before 34 weeks), if the delivery is complicated and instruments are used, if you are too tired from your efforts so far, or if the baby is in distress and the birth is imminent.

Without an episiotomy many women will suffer tears in the skin and the superficial muscles guarding the entrance to the vagina, but episiotomies are often more extensive than required. Furthermore, an episiotomy may deprive you of the internal sensations that help you to push your baby out. (For more details about coping with an episiotomy, see p. 120.)

Cutting the cord　　Some obstetricians advocate that the cord should be allowed to stop pulsating before it is cut, to give the baby as much oxygenated blood as possible, but it is still common for the umbilical cord to be cut very soon after the baby is born. Then the midwife usually sucks the baby's nose and mouth clear of mucus and fluid.

The third stage of labour

To cut down the amount of blood that is lost when the placenta separates, it is usual to give you an injection of a mixture of ergometrine and oxytocin (Syntometrine) just as the baby is about to be born. The placenta should then separate with the birth of the baby so that it follows the baby's bottom to rest in the cervix and upper vagina, and can then be delivered almost immediately. This is most often done by the method of cord traction and supra-pubic pressure: which means that the midwife takes the cord in one hand and with the other presses on the abdomen to steady the uterus. By pulling the cord down she draws the placenta out of the vagina. If nature is left to herself, you can push the placenta out yourself. Suckling the baby at the breast also causes the uterus to contract and to expel the placenta.

Complications

Any section on complicated labours is going to sound rather pessimistic and grim. As you read this, remember that statistically the chances are that your labour will be quite straightforward. However, since one never knows in advance what kind of labour is in store, it is best to learn about the common complications so that if you do happen to experience one or more of them you will be prepared and better able to cope.

Induction of labour

There are good reasons why labour sometimes needs to be induced, such as raised blood pressure (toxaemia), diabetes, Rhesus incompatibility, and bleeding in late pregnancy. The reasons for induction should be explained to you and your willing consent to the operation should be obtained.

Many obstetricians do not like women to go past the expected date of delivery by more than a few days, and/or they like to induce labour if the diastolic blood pressure (the second figure of the recorded level, e.g. 130/95) exceeds 90 mm of mercury. However, other obstetricians doubt whether, if the mother is otherwise healthy, these are by themselves sufficient justifications to induce labour. If you are not satisfied with the reason given to you, you should insist on a further explanation.

If labour is to be induced, you may be asked to stay in hospital the night before the induction is planned. The next morning you will go through the ritual of pubic shave, enema, and bath. If your cervix is 'ripe' (soft, short, beginning to open, and the baby's head is in the pelvic cavity) labour may be induced by rupturing the membranes. You will be asked to empty your bladder and then to lie on a delivery bed with your hips and knees bent, your feet supported in stirrups and your legs apart. This is the lithotomy position. The doctor washes your vulva down with an antiseptic solution, confirms the state of the cervix and the position of the baby by a vaginal examination, and then nicks a hole in the membranes bulging through the cervix (forewaters) with a pair of forceps passed along his fingers.

If the cervix is not ripe, induction is usually brought about by putting a needle into a vein in your arm so that a solution containing the hormone oxytocin can be dripped into your circulation at a controlled rate to make your uterus contract and open the cervix. Later on the membranes can be ruptured.

Some obstetricians always combine rupture of the membranes with the use of intravenous oxytocin to induce labour. Prostaglandin tablets or creams are sometimes used in the vagina to ripen the cervix as a preparation for induction, or as a means of inducing labour.

Bleeding in labour

Labour usually starts with a show of blood, which is the thick, sticky mucus plug from the cervix with some fresh or older blood. Continued fresh bleeding, however, is not normal. The reason for this may be that the placenta is placed abnormally low in the uterus (placenta praevia) and below the leading part of the baby. Under these circumstances the baby can only be born safely by delivery from above the placenta using Caesarian section.

If abnormal bleeding occurs when labour has begun and the position of the placenta is not already known from an ultrasound scan examination, a vaginal examination is made in an operating theatre, with preparations complete for Caesarean section, to feel whether or not the placenta is in the way. Depending on the degree of likelihood of placenta praevia being present, and therefore the need for a Caesarean section, you may be given a general anaesthetic for this examination.

Foetal distress

Foetal distress means that the baby is suffering from lack of oxygen. Warning that this may be happening is given by the passage of meconium from the baby's bowels so that the amniotic fluid is stained green or yellow, and by changes in the foetal heart-rate outside the normal limits of 120 to 160 beats per minute. If these warning signs occur, a foetal heart-rate monitor can be used to make a continuous recording of what is happening.

If evidence of foetal distress persists or gets worse, action is usually taken to deliver the baby as soon as possible. If foetal distress occurs in the first stage of labour, before the cervix is fully dilated, Caesarean section is necessary. If it happens in the second stage of labour, depending on the position of the baby's head, delivery may be hastened by an episiotomy or by using forceps.

Some obstetricians will give you oxygen to breathe if signs of foetal distress appear or will ask you to lie on your side, since this increases the blood flow to the uterus. In some hospitals a sample of the baby's blood is obtained for gas analysis to find out whether the signs of foetal distress are caused by lack of oxygen or by another reason. This foetal blood sample is taken with you in the lithotomy position. A metal tube (amnioscope) is passed along the vagina and through the cervix to prick the baby's head. The drip of blood that oozes out is sucked up in a tube so that it can be analysed.

Prolapse of the umbilical cord   Foetal distress may also occur, and usually very suddenly, if the umbilical cord slips down and is compressed against your pelvic bones. The time when this is most likely to happen is when the waters break before the baby's head is engaged in the pelvis. If the cervix is not fully dilated, the baby can be delivered by Caesarean section. In the second stage of labour, the birth can be hurried along by making an episiotomy or by using forceps.

Cord entanglement   It is quite common for the umbilical cord to be looped loosely around the baby's body or neck. More rarely the cord is shortened so much by the entanglement that during contractions, particularly in the second stage, it may be pulled tight so that blood is unable to flow freely to the baby, causing distress. At delivery, if the cord is looped around the neck of the baby, it is usually quite easy to slip the baby through the loops. Otherwise, a tight cord can be cut between clamps, to stop it bleeding and free the baby.

Cephalo-pelvic disproportion

Disproportion means that the baby's head is too big to pass easily through the mother's bony pelvis, because the baby is too big, because the head is relatively larger than it should be, or because her pelvis is too small. This possibility may have been suspected before labour from your small stature, examination of the pelvis, or because the baby's head does not engage in your pelvis. The size of the baby's head can be measured using ultrasound, and the size of your pelvis can be measured on an X-ray. With disproportion, progress in labour is slow and may cease. The only safe way to deal with this problem is by Caesarean section. If disproportion is suspected but not absolutely certain before your labour begins, a trial of labour may be conducted to see whether the baby can negotiate the birth canal reasonably, but everything will be ready to do a Ceasarean operation should it prove necessary.

Abnormal positions of the head

In normal birth the top of the baby's head (the vertex) is the first part to appear. The baby has his chin tucked well into his chest so that he looks backwards to your spine and the back of his head lies towards your abdomen (occipito-anterior position). Sometimes, however, the baby's head is not in this usual position and steps must be taken to assist the birth.

Occipito-posterior positions   When labour begins the back of the baby's head (occiput) usually points to one or other side, and only turns to the front as labour progresses and the head gets lower in the pelvis. Sometimes the back of the baby's head rotates towards your spine instead of forwards: this is an occipito-posterior position, and often means that labour is prolonged and that contractions tend to be less regular and to be associated with a lot of backache. In most women who start labour with an occipito-posterior position, rotation forwards does occur and the baby is delivered normally.

If the occipito-posterior position persists, the baby can still be delivered normally with his face looking towards your abdomen, a so-called 'face-to-pubes' delivery. On some occasions the baby's head fails to rotate completely and progress in the second stage is slowed right down because the baby's head can turn neither backwards nor forwards – it is stuck looking side-ways (deep transverse arrest). This situation requires correction and delivery under anaesthesia by turning the baby's head with a hand, with forceps, or with the vacuum extractor (Ventouse).

Problems of head flexion   If the baby's head is not well tucked into his chest (i.e. not fully flexed on the spine), the baby's head is not as small as it can be to pass down the birth canal. This may result in delay in labour, especially in the second stage. If deflexion occurs in the second stage – usually with an occipito-posterior position or deep transverse arrest – it is corrected at the same time as the fault in rotation, under anaesthesia. If the baby's head becomes still more deflexed so that the forehead is leading to give a *brow presentation*, labour is completely obstructed and delivery by Caesarean section is necessary. This is a very rare complication. More commonly, but still rarely, the baby's head is completely unbent on the spine so that the face actually leads and looks down the birth canal. *Face presentations* can be delivered normally although assis-tance may be necessary. Because the face takes all the pressure of labour, at birth it is swollen and bruised. This passes off within three to four days and leaves the baby without permanent damage and looking normal.

Breech presentation

Ninety-eight per cent of babies in the last few weeks before delivery settle to lie head downwards and are born this way. In the remainder the bottom or breech of the baby is the present-ing part. Breech deliveries cause concern because the risks of delivery for the baby are greater than if the head comes first. This is because the head is the largest part of the baby and it has the most difficulty in passing through the pelvis. In normal labour the head has a long time to adapt and mould itself, whereas in breech delivery the head has to pass through the birth canal in a matter of a few minutes. This means that there is more chance of damage inside the baby's head if it passes through too quickly, whilst if there is delay in the birth of the head there is a greater chance that the baby will suffer from lack of oxygen.

For a breech delivery to be safe, therefore, the pelvis must be roomy. To be certain of this, X-ray pelvimetry (pelvic measurement) may be helpful, to find out whether vaginal delivery or Caesarean section would be the safer method of birth.

Because of the risks of breech delivery, some doctors try to turn babies so that they are head down before labour starts – *external cephalic version*. Others think that you succeed in turning only those who would have turned by themselves anyway.

The first stage of labour is the same whether the head or breech presents. In the second stage, help and anaesthesia are more often required.

Twins

With two or more babies labour usually starts a week or two before the expected date of delivery. The first stage is as usual. The babies may be born head or breech first in almost any combination. There is usually a pause of 10–20 minutes between the birth of one baby and the next. The placenta is delivered after both babies.

Transverse lie

Rarely labour may start with the baby lying across your abdomen instead of either head or breech first. He cannot be delivered like this and so Caesarean section is usually required, unless before the membranes rupture he can be turned easily and nothing (like the placenta) is obstructing the pelvis.

Unstable lie

Some babies even near the expected date of delivery may constantly change their position from head to breech presentations to transverse lie. This sort of unstable lie is dangerous because it may be the result of obstruction to the birth canal, which requires special treatment. An unstable lie is also more likely to be associated with prolapse of the umbilical cord when the membranes rupture. For these reasons women with an unstable lie are often observed in hospital until the baby is born so that any unexpected complications can be dealt with immediately.

Forceps delivery

When the baby is presenting by the head, forceps are used to hasten delivery if there is foetal distress, if you become too tired or distressed, or if progress is too slow. Most obstetricians would regard two hours as the upper limit for a normal second stage in a first labour, and one hour if you are having your second or subsequent baby. Some obstetricians are more active than this and may regard half that time as long enough.

Anaesthesia is required for forceps delivery: either general anaesthesia, epidural anaesthesia, or pudendal block. Pudendal block is local anaesthetic injected around the vulva and into the vagina to numb the nerves supplying these parts. An episiotomy is usually done to make forceps delivery easier so that it causes less damage to your tissues and less force is applied to the baby.

Manual removal of the placenta

The placenta is usually delivered within 30 minutes of your baby's birth. If there is delay beyond this, or if at any time heavy bleeding occurs, the placenta can be removed by the doctor. A general anaesthetic is given (if you do not already have an epidural) and the doctor passes a hand along the vagina and into the uterus to separate the placenta with his fingers and then remove it.

How to cope with a Caesarean section

Some women need a surgical operation called a 'Caesarean section' to deliver their babies. If your doctor suggests during your antenatal care that a Caesarean section may be advisable, discuss this fully. Many couples want to be fully informed, to share in the decision-making and, if necessary, to ask for a second obstetric opinion. Sometimes, however, a Caesarean must be done for an unexpected reason, so it is worth knowing about Caesareans, even if you probably won't have one.

There are many possible reasons for a Caesarean birth: some can be diagnosed well in advance, such as cephalo-pelvic disproportion (where the baby's head is too big to be delivered through the mother's pelvis); others, such as foetal distress (when the baby is suffering from lack of oxygen) or placenta praevia (where the afterbirth is over the cervix), may not be recognized until labour has started. Sometimes when a Caesarean will probably be needed, but is not absolutely indicated, a woman may be allowed to go into labour spontaneously or have her labour induced to see whether a normal birth is possible. Everything will be ready to do a Caesarean operation if necessary.

The operation

A Caesarean section operation involves cutting through the mother's abdomen (under anaesthetic, of course) to enable the doctor to lift the baby directly out of the uterus instead of letting it be born through the vagina. It is a major operation after which the mother and baby will need special care and attention, and a hospital stay of ten days or so is inevitable.

If the operation is planned (rather than an emergency) you may be given some premedication so you feel drowsy on your way to the theatre; conversely, the anaesthetist may decide to minimize the use of drugs for the baby's sake. Discuss this with your doctor so you know what to expect.

In the operating theatre, the anaesthetist will give you an injection and possibly a mask to breathe through, which he may let you hold. Usually a catheter is passed to drain the bladder so that it will not be in the way. Relaxing the pelvic floor helps you to cope if this is done before the anaesthetic.

The baby is usually delivered within five to ten minutes. The paediatrician looks after the baby while the obstetrician delivers the placenta and closes the incision in the uterus and the abdominal wall. The abdomen is closed with metal clips (removed by about the seventh day) or with black silk or nylon sutures. The whole operation may take twenty to thirty minutes.

Your abdominal scar may be horizontal or vertical, and is usually six to nine inches long. A bikini will cover a horizontal scar.

Helping yourself and the baby

Even if you know you are going to have a Caesarean section, attending antenatal classes and practising for a normal delivery is still well worthwhile. You will learn how your body works during pregnancy, and the exercises, relaxation, and breathing techniques will be useful before and after the baby is born. Some women feel that 'labour rehearsals', done in class, are some substitute for the experience they will miss.

If the operation is an emergency and your labour is already under way, it is tempting to stop bothering to cope with contractions once the need for a Caesarean is announced; but you should continue to use your breathing and relaxation so that the baby receives the maximum oxygen.

To prepare for the time after the operation, try getting in and out of bed and chairs, and positioning the baby (use a pillow) for feeds as described below. Practise this special breathing exercise for use after the operation to rid your lungs of general anaesthetic. Place your hands on the sides of your lower ribs, breathe out with a little hiss for as long as you can, feeling your hands come together as you do it. Then breathe in, letting your ribs expand sideways. Repeat four times; then take a deep breath in, let the breath out quickly, and cough as deeply as possible.

You and your baby will be healthier if you stop smoking during pregnancy, and your recovery will be quicker.

Your husband may be disappointed if he cannot be present at the birth, but he may be with you until you enter the theatre, and can perhaps be there when you come round from the anaesthetic to tell you about the baby. This can help you both, and you can welcome the baby together.

Epidural anaesthesia

It may be possible for you to have an epidural so that you are fully conscious for the operation. In this case you would be numb in the area of the abdomen but be able to hear your baby's first cry and see him as soon as he is born. The surgeon may also agree for your husband to be present.

After the operation

The baby often recovers quickly, and can be put into his father's arms even before you regain consciousness. In some cases, however, the baby may be in a special care unit for a time. If he cannot come to see you, the staff will usually take you to see him. If you know in advance that the operation is to be performed, you could discuss this with the paediatrician beforehand.

Touch the baby as soon as you can and cuddle him. He may be drowsy from your general anaesthetic, but this should wear off after a few days.

Your abdomen will be sore and you may suffer from wind. Moving about as much as possible, in bed or out, will help this. There may also be some bladder discomfort from the catheter. When you get out of bed, the footstool or chair is often helpful, especially if the bed is high.

You may need painkilling drugs like pethidine for the first 48 hours, so breastfeeding may not be allowed during this time. But you should start getting yourself mobile to help your recovery and the healing of the scar.

It is very important to breathe the remains of any anaesthetic out of your lungs and to cough up any mucus which may be present. Do the breathing exercise described earlier as soon as you come round, but cup your hands under your abdomen to support it, or hold a pillow against it, when you try to cough. A physiotherapist will probably be available to help you get the breathing right and may assist the coughing by tapping your chest. Coughing will not open your wound and will prevent chest complications. Support the scar if you are going to sneeze or laugh, and relax to prevent your body tensing up and increasing the pain.

Getting up

Push your palms into the bed close to your sides and lift your bottom. Repeat this until you reach the side of the bed. With both hands lift your outside leg at the knee and place your foot on the footstool or floor, then repeat with the inside knee, so that you can ease yourself out of bed. Do not try to lift a whole leg from the hip. Or you can shift your legs to the side of the bed by waggling one foot sideways (heel-toes, heel-toes) and then doing the same with the other until your legs are together, then sit upright on the edge of the bed. However you do it, *take your time, breathe long, slow, gentle breaths, and do everything yourself*. When asked to get out of bed during bed-making, remember these guidelines and don't let someone unwittingly hurt you by wrong lifting.

Getting into bed

Vertical scar   Face the side of the bed, climb on to the footstool and then on to the bed on all fours, turn and 'reverse' well up back against the pillows. Inching your way sideways is slower and more uncomfortable.

Horizontal scar   Sit well back on to the bed with your back against the pillows, slowly lift and slide your legs on to the bed one at a time, and lift your bottom into the pillows by pushing down with your palms.

After a few days, if you slip down and need propping up, you can hold on to the bar above to take the strain while you tuck your bottom against the pillows. Dig your heels into the sheets.

Walking

Stand up straight so that gravity does not pull the weight of your abdominal contents against the scar. Support your abdomen and, using the breathing you learned for labour, move from bed to chair as though this were a contraction. Calm breathing is helpful to relax you before feeding and after walking or moving about.

Sitting

Choose hard, upright chairs, if possible with arms. To sit, take hold of the arms, put one leg behind the other, bend your knees to take the strain, then sit. Reverse this to get up. If your chair has no arms, sit on one buttock, while holding on to the chair back, and edge back sideways.

Using the lavatory

Again, use bent knees to take the strain of sitting down, and hold on to any rails nearby. Relax your pelvic floor and the muscles of your face (which are associated with the pelvic floor muscles) to help the flow of urine. You may need a laxative.

Washing

A bidet may be available. You may find this easier to use than climbing into a bath and it may feel safer than standing in a shower. Whichever you use, remember to check the temperature of the water before you start. Use the bidet to wash your feet as well: they are very hard to reach otherwise!

Breastfeeding

Your milk may be a little late coming in (it has been known to take as long as 10–12 days), but the baby should still be put to the breast and a complement of water or formula offered afterwards if the paediatrician thinks it necessary. This will help to stimulate your milk supply and it will soon become properly established.

As your abdomen is sore, special feeding positions may be necessary. Use conscious relaxation and smiling to help with the discomfort and after-pains.

If you have a vertical scar   (a) Put a pillow on one side of you and rest the baby's head on it with his feet over your thighs. This means there is less strain involved in holding the baby up. (b) Lay the baby on a pillow with his head facing the breast and feed him lying under your arm. Sit straight to avoid straining your abdomen.

Feeding position after a Caesarean – vertical scar

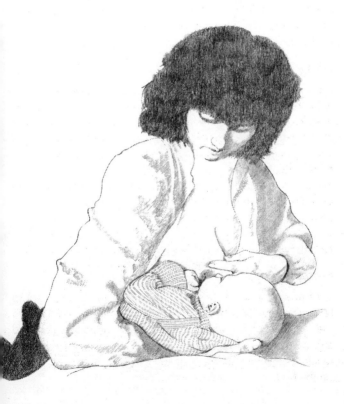

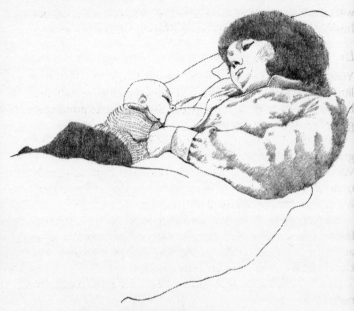

Feeding position after a Caesarean – horizontal scar

If you have a horizontal scar   (a) Lay pillows horizontally across your stomach and feed normally. (b) Lie down on the bed on your side with the baby beside you and feed him facing you.

Possible difficulties

Sometimes after a Caesarean it is difficult to realize that the baby in the cot beside you is the 'bump' you have had for the last nine months. Breastfeeding can be a real help in this situation, building up your relationship and making you feel certain that this is your baby. But even if you bottle-feed, you can help make this 'your baby' in lots of other ways. Talk to the baby: tell him about his home and his family. Lie with him against your bare skin if you can. Not every mother falls in love with her new baby at first sight; it may take time. Do not feel guilty if you feel detached about the baby; this can happen with any type of birth experience. Confiding your fears to your husband may help; he may well be feeling the same way!

Living in hospital

Your stay in hospital will probably be about ten days. It can be a little disheartening when others are going home after 48 hours, but you need the extra care and rest. Use the time to advantage getting to know your baby.

Dispense with the back-rest at night as soon as possible and gradually learn to sleep with your normal number of pillows. When you first turn on your side, one or two pillows partly under your abdomen and partly under your upper flexed knee will provide support, particularly to a vertical scar.

You will have a lochia (a discharge from the uterus rather like a menstrual period) as with a vaginal birth. Soft stretch pants are much more comfortable than sanitary belts. Loose soft clothes with no front zips are best.

Use your postnatal exercises to help your figure return to normal.

Your husband

A new father with his wife and baby in hospital, even for 48 hours, is likely to feel lonely and extra busy with work, hospital visits, shopping, and shouldering new responsibilities. A husband whose wife and baby are in hospital for an extended time after a Caesarean (whether expected or not) will probably feel even more strongly that he is an outsider. He may miss his wife and worry that visiting times are so short that he cannot give her the emotional support she needs. He may not have as much contact with the baby as he would wish, and may feel remote from his new child. He may be concerned that the conception of the baby was his responsibility and that he has 'caused' pain to his wife. He may also have practical problems with cooking, and the care of his other children. Most friends and relatives are only too pleased to be asked to help out at this time, and he should not feel embarrassed to approach them. His wife should not concentrate so much on her own problems that she cannot recognize his; they should give one another loving support where it is needed.

The future

Ask the medical or nursing staff if you have any queries. Find out exactly why you needed a Caesarean section so that you can tell another doctor the next time you are pregnant. Some doctors say that after a Caesarean you should wait at least one year before becoming pregnant again; some advocate no more than three Caesareans. If the same complications recur in a subsequent pregnancy it may be necessary to have another Caesarean section, but if everything appears straightforward then the next baby may be born normally. For your safety it will, however, be necessary for any later deliveries to take place in a consultant hospital – not a nursing home or a GP unit.

Episiotomy

Episiotomy is the surgical enlargement of the birth outlet, used to prevent over-stretching of the pelvic floor and to enable the baby to be born easily and without tearing the muscles of the mother's pelvic floor. In some hospitals episiotomies are routine with first babies. However, a mother who can relax her pelvic floor and work with the midwife during the delivery of her baby is less likely to need an episiotomy than a mother who is tense.

Some doctors and midwives feel that far too many routine episiotomies are done nowadays. Until the last decade or so, midwives were taught to deliver babies so that episiotomies were rare and a mother's intact perineum was a tribute to the midwife's skill. Then episiotomies became medically fashionable to prevent damage to the mother's tissues, to avoid later prolapse of the uterus, and to give a 'nice tight vagina' for subsequent sexual intercourse. The pendulum is swinging again and there are doctors who now believe that a second degree tear is often preferable to an episiotomy, because the tear is limited by need and not by the judgement of the midwife or obstetrician who is making the cut with a pair of scissors. They feel that prolapses are less common now that women are better fed and have fewer children, and that some episiotomies are performed with inadequate anaesthesia and repaired badly.

There are, obviously, cases where episiotomy is very necessary for the sake of both mother and baby. But it is a good idea, at your antenatal visits, to discuss your hospital's policy about episiotomy and make your own views known to those who will be taking care of you. Tell them again when you are in labour.

What to do before the baby is born

Suitable exercises which increase the voluntary control of the muscles and increase the blood supply to the pelvic floor to improve its condition and healing property are:

Tighten and relax the muscles controlling the passage of urine (practise this while urinating).

Tighten and relax the ring of muscles around the anus.

Raise and lower the pelvic floor, imagining it to be a lift in a building, slowly going up, going down again, down into the basement (bulging out the vagina) and drawing up to the ground floor again.

Make smooth movements with the vaginal muscles, as though rolling them around a tennis ball (clockwise and then counter-clockwise); or imagine writing or drawing with a pencil held in the vagina.

(Note: the latter sets of exercises need not involve any movement of the thigh muscles – the legs should be slightly apart and the exercises may be practised while sitting, lying, standing, or kneeling.)

Practise the delivery position, half-lying with your upper back and head supported on several pillows, knees bent with the feet resting on the bed, hip-width apart and with the knees allowed to flop outwards. Sit with the weight on the base of your spine, not on your buttocks.

Practising for the delivery of the baby's head and shoulders should be done with relaxed thigh muscles and mouth, to help relax the vagina. Smiling helps many people to relax.

The episiotomy

A local anaesthetic will be given in advance if it is obvious that an episiotomy will be needed, since it takes several minutes before the tissues are numbed. If it is done during delivery to prevent tearing, the cut is made at the peak of a contraction when the nerve endings are numbed by the stretching. In either case, the mother should be aware only of stretching caused by the pressure of the baby's head and then sudden relief as the episiotomy enlarges the opening and the baby's head slips out. If it is done as an emergency procedure it may not be possible to ensure the mother's comfort, but she can reassure herself that although it hurt, it was done quickly and to help her and her baby.

After an episiotomy, stitching will be necessary. More local anaesthetic should be given especially if there is a delay in suturing. If the stitching is painful, you should tell the doctor and say that the anaesthetic has not yet taken effect. If only one or two stitches are necessary you may be offered gas and oxygen rather than an injection.

Coping with the stitches

Some kinds of stitches dissolve after five or six days, others need to be removed when the cut has healed, again usually after five or six days. Some mothers experience few problems with stitches. However, for those who are uncomfortable or bruised, the following suggestions may be helpful.

Lie on your tummy, or half-lie on your back or side; it may be easier than sitting. For relief of discomfort, some hospitals recommend frequent warm salt baths; some suggest using a bidet; still others suggest swabbing the pelvic area.

Sit well back on the lavatory: this helps to prevent urine stinging sore tissues. Hold the stitched area firmly with a clean pad when opening your bowels. Use soft toilet paper rather than hard (take your own to hospital if necessary).

Wear a sanitary belt to hold your pads, since this will provide firmer support than the sanitary pants into which pads can be inserted. Pants allow movement of the pad as you walk, and this will rub the stitches. Self-adhesive pads will also rub in this way. Once the stitches have been removed, it may also be far more comfortable to use two-layer, soft paper-filled sanitary pads rather than the harsher paper-cotton wool types.

Some mothers find homoeopathic arnica tablets helpful; lanolin-based homoeopathic arnica ointment or hypercal ointment or tincture can be applied to the stitched area to reduce bruising.

For breastfeeding, you may find side-lying the most comfortable position; if your underneath elbow is raised on a pillow, it is easier for the baby to feed from the nipple. Take care to see that your breast is not compressed against the chest-wall, as this may lead to engorgement. Other suggestions for comfortable breastfeeding are to sit in an upright chair or to sit upright in bed with the baby on a pillow under your arm.

Healing

A carefully stitched episiotomy should heal neatly, though you may find it very tender and painful for the first week, and occasionally uncomfortable for some weeks or even months after that.

Pelvic floor exercises should be started as soon as possible after the birth, and repeated frequently each day. After the delivery you can practise stream-stopping when passing urine, and gentle up-and-down movements of the whole pelvic floor, at any time. As the soreness decreases you can isolate the muscle movements and increase them in strength. Emphasis should now be put on tightening the muscles around the vagina and holding them tight for a count of four before relaxing.

You may find it reassuring to look at the pelvic floor with a hand mirror before the birth to see that there is space for the incision, and afterwards to see how small an area has been stitched.

Making love again

The problems of making love after an episiotomy are discussed on p. 202, but to sum up:

There is no magical date after which it is 'all right' to make love. The ideal time is when both partners desire it, regardless of the baby's age. Your pelvic floor muscles may be sore or tight following stitches, but waiting will not make them stretch. Your husband may be just as afraid of hurting you as you are afraid of being hurt; plenty of love-play before intercourse, with each having consideration for the other, helps to dispel any fear. Lubrication with special creams or jellies will make penetration more comfortable.

Bonding – developing early relationships with the baby

Bonding is the word which has recently been used to describe the developing relationship between mothers – or fathers – and their newborn babies. This relationship is a two-way process: the baby learning to respond to his parents, and the parents to the child. It has been compared to courtship, it goes on over a long period of time, and it is unique to each pair of people. Many of its aspects are unlike any other human relationship, but there are also features which are not so different from a relationship, say, between a man and a woman in love.

What do parents want to know about bonding? What do they need to know about it? Chiefly, perhaps, to trust their own feelings.

Nearly every woman finds that as soon as her baby is born,

she wants to hold him and to see and touch, at last, the baby which has been a part of her for so many months. The classic sketch of parents counting their baby's fingers and toes has always been a source of amusement, but it reflects a real and natural impulse, and parents who have been unable to hold their babies soon after birth have often felt unhappy about it at the time and for long afterwards. Some mothers who have held one child soon after its birth but had another child taken away, for whatever reason, have felt that it was easier for them to feel a sense of 'belonging' with the child held early than with the child taken away.

Recent research has demonstrated that this long-held feeling about the value of early holding of the newborn baby by his mother is founded on a good basis of fact. Research has been done, for instance, which suggests that the first hour and a half after a baby is born is a time of particular sensitivity and alertness in mother and baby, and that if the baby and its mother are not together during any of this time, then it may take extra effort for the 'bonding' process to proceed. Interest in this field of research arose from animal research (some mammals actually reject their offspring if not given contact immediately, although this is not true of human beings) and has been followed by careful research with human beings. This showed in particular that mothers who held their babies for an hour as soon as they were born and for extra time (in comparison with the other mothers in the study) on each of the next few days, established close relationships with their babies sooner than mothers given less contact. Two years later the mothers who had experienced extended contact used more questions, more adjectives and fewer commands, and at five years old their children scored better on language tests.

This kind of research has helped all those working in maternity and paediatric care, or interested in parent-child relationships, to make it easier for the bonding process to begin, and to give special help in the cases where the mother and baby must be separated. It should be stressed that bonding is not something that has to be *done to* mothers and babies, but that it is a part of the process by which the new life assimilates the world. It is part of the long journey from fertilized egg to independent individual and ought not to be disrupted. Hospital routines which put babies into nurseries for almost all the time and bring them to their mothers only for clock-controlled feedtimes are an example of patterns to avoid: fortunately this attitude towards the care of mothers and babies is less widespread than it once was. Of course the mother should not become over-tired, but she should be able to be with her baby as much as she likes and to share the baby with her husband, too.

Pregnancy

When a woman becomes pregnant there are things about her that will affect how she will behave with her baby: such things as her genetic inheritance from her own parents, her upbringing and education, her relationship with the child's father, and her beliefs about child-rearing practices. These and other factors will influence – and be influenced by – her actual experiences during pregnancy, labour, delivery, and then living with the baby.

Love between two adult individuals can be a mixture of many emotions, just as it can be between parents and children. The love of a parent for a child encompasses many facets including tenderness, protectiveness, and a powerful sense of belonging. Not all these emotions may be aroused at once, and there seems to be a great variation in when mothers first feel love for their babies. Some feel it first in pregnancy itself (especially when they first feel the baby move), some at the baby's birth, and some during the first few weeks after delivery. (The father, too, may find that his love does not come instantly, but grows and develops as he and the baby get to know one another.) The feelings of mother-love in pregnancy may be mingled with other feelings, such as fear or anxiety about whether the baby will be perfect.

During pregnancy there are already strong influences

between the mother and her baby: hormonal changes caused by the baby's presence alter the mother's physiology, emotions, and behaviour. Her behaviour and emotions will in turn affect the baby's behaviour, probably via further hormones crossing from her blood across the placenta to the baby. External things will also influence the baby's behaviour inside the uterus: the sound of the blood flow through her uterus, loud noises, alterations in her position, light getting across the thin wall of her abdomen and uterus – all these will be appreciated by the unborn child. Perhaps – but this is not yet proved – the baby towards the end of pregnancy has already grown familiar with some aspects of her, such as the individual rhythms and variations of her heart-beat, which he may remember after birth.

Birth and afterwards

A woman's experience of childbirth is also likely to affect how her relationship with her baby develops, although this is not a matter of simple cause and effect: even the most strenuous, unusual, or painful labour can be the beginning of a firm 'bonding' if the mother makes it as positive an experience as she can.

Immediately after birth, particularly if no pain-killing drugs have been given, the mother and baby appear to go through a period of especial alertness lasting up to an hour and a half. It would seem natural that as far as possible, mothers, fathers, and babies should be together in close contact during this time. The baby in the mother's arms has the advantage of being warm and being kept near the breast. If he suckles the breast, he will aid the let-down reflex and help with the third stage of labour. The baby will also be near the comforting sound of the mother's heartbeat, and by being in close contact with her will be beginning to learn new features about her: her face, her voice, her smell, and her behaviour. From the parent's point of view this early contact with their baby may help them in their developing relationships with the child, and may have influences on their behaviour later on. For this reason – that it may in some way facilitate their relationship – mothers should be helped to have early contact with their babies whenever possible. It is not essential, however, and where a very small or sick baby has to be taken away to have further care, the immediate health of the baby is of prime importance. After all, most relationships of any kind suffer temporary setbacks but are picked up again and developed at a later stage, ideally with the help of those around and concerned.

For human beings there is obviously no right or wrong way to behave with a baby immediately after birth, and from observations done in delivery rooms and at home births, there is every kind of variation. However, there do appear to be some kinds of behaviour which occur more often than others. For instance, there is a tendency for the mother to touch the baby first with her finger-tips – very gently and tentatively – then to stroke the baby with her fingers, and then to manipulate the limbs. There also appears to be an interest in the baby's eyes, with verbal encouragement to open them, and then a direct greeting of the baby when he does. Some mothers have reported that they do not really feel that the baby is alive until he has opened his eyes. Many mothers in this period also compare some feature of the baby with the baby's father, if he is present.

What of the baby during these moments? He may not go through such a long period of alertness for several further days. If he is in his mother's arms he may gaze into her face, for the newborn baby is particularly responsive to the features of human beings and, held in this position, his face is about nine inches away from his mother's face – the distance at which he can see best. He is also responsive to the sound of the human voice, especially slightly higher frequencies, which may explain why people tend to raise the pitch of their voices when talking to babies.

The first few months

Over the first weeks and months, the parents and the baby continue to learn, understand, and respond to one another's needs. The mother has to develop a new pattern of responsibility, covering 24 hours a day of feeding, cuddling, changing, cleaning, and talking to her child – and an infinite number of other responses. The father likewise finds that his role changes. It has been shown that fathers who are present at their children's births and who help to look after their babies immediately after birth, continue to offer support and practical help with care, almost as if they too have become bonded.

The baby, meanwhile, is learning about his parents. By six days of age he is able to distinguish between the smell of his own mother and the smell of a stranger; by ten days he seems able to distinguish between the caring ways of his own mother and those of a stranger. At three weeks of age he will respond differently to the sight of his own mother's face and to the sound of her voice, than to the face and voice of a stranger. Thus even this early, the baby – having been born with the ability to be more attracted to human beings than to objects in the environment – has become even more specific and has learned to respond particularly to his own parents: in fact, he has become bonded to them.

If separation does occur

Sometimes separation of the mother and baby is unavoidable: special care of mother or baby may be required, for instance, if the birth has been long or complicated, if an assisted delivery or Caesarean section has been required, or if the baby is ill or premature. It is important in such cases to remember that these mothers and babies will nevertheless develop their own relationship, starting whenever they can, and that some initial separation is not an irreparable 'bad start'. The bonding process is best facilitated by enabling mother and baby to have as much time together as possible, as soon as possible, but in human beings it is fortunately not absolutely dependent on a particular time or pattern. If you and your baby must be separated, do not be discouraged but do make every opportunity to be together, to look at the baby, to help with his care whenever possible, and to begin the bonding process as soon as you can, giving extra attention then in cuddles, holding, talking, singing, rocking, relaxing, and feeding. If the separation is to be prolonged, you may like to take a hint from one special care baby unit which gives each mother a photograph of her baby to keep with her while the baby is in special care.

It is also helpful to remember that new parents and babies are often rather shy of each other at first – whether the first contact is immediately at the baby's birth or delayed somewhat – and need to allow themselves time to get to know each other. Just as some friendships start very quickly, like 'falling in love at first sight', and some others take longer to form, like a good wine maturing or a green fruit ripening, so some parents very quickly feel a powerful sense of connection with their babies, while others develop this feeling more slowly. Many factors are involved, and there is no magic formula which results in instant bonding, nor any hard-and-fast rules which must be followed, nor even any typical pattern: you and your baby will form, given time together, a special relationship which is yours alone.

THE NEW
BABY

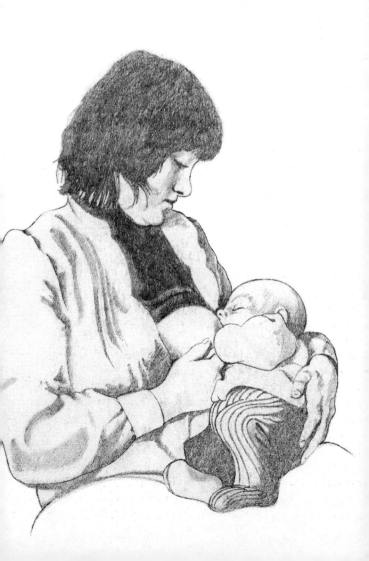

Introduction

Watching your baby grow and develop new skills is one of the most rewarding pleasures of parenthood, although of course it is wrong to be so obsessed with the next milestone that you ignore present achievements. We are recognizing how many skills even newborn babies possess, and they are no longer written off as helpless and passive little creatures.

Breastfeeding can be the most convenient and mutually satisfying way of feeding a baby. If you decide to breastfeed, it will be helpful for you to learn the theory beforehand. It would be reasonable to suppose that breastfeeding comes instinctively to the mother, but this does not necessarily happen. For thousands of years women have watched one another feeding babies and have learned, perhaps unconsciously, how it was done: what positions were most comfortable, what to do when there were physical snags, and so on. In one British community it was the custom for nursing mothers to wear a blue thread which had been handed down from mother to daughter through several generations. Ostensibly this was to ward off mastitis, but it must have acted as a tangible moral support: 'If my mother can do it, so can I.' However, nowadays the sight of a nursing mother is quite rare and women are thrown back on to their own resources to find out about the process of lactation.

If, for some reason, you cannot breastfeed your baby, or do not wish to do so, feel confident that the artificial milks available today are more satisfactory than their predecessors were. Whatever method of feeding you choose, the most important thing is to ensure that feedtimes are loving and happy occasions.

When your baby is about six months old he will probably like to start a mixed diet of milk and solids. It is quite unnecessary to spend a lot of money on commercially-prepared baby food (other than for convenience) since the baby can easily eat modified versions of the family's meals.

This book does not set out to tell you exactly how to care for your baby, since the way you choose to do this will be individual to you, your personality and your circumstances. A few general hints, however, may apply to most people.

Some parents have specialized problems, if their babies are born prematurely or are handicapped in some way. Modern paediatric medicine can now do a great deal to help these children.

The parents of twins have to cope with the mixed blessings of a 'package-deal family' and may find it helpful to discover how best to cut corners and adapt their lives to the extra demands twin babies make.

Adoptive parents require information about infant feeding and basic babycare, too, and have special emotional needs as well, particularly during the period before the adoption is finalized.

The development of your baby from birth to one year old

Is it all right?' is the first question asked by most new parents.

The midwife (or doctor, if there is one present) is concerned first to ascertain that your baby's head, spine, and limbs appear normal, and this is done at a glance. At the same time she will check to see that breathing begins within a minute or so and that the baby is a good colour, indicating that the heart and circulation are going well. She will also see that he is lively and that his muscle 'tone' is not too floppy. Sometimes the condition of the baby is rated by Apgar score (named after the doctor who devised it), in which each of five headings is checked and given a score of 0, 1, or 2; they are heart-rate, respiratory effort, muscle tone, colour, and reflex irritability, and the maximum score of 10 indicates a truly lusty babe. The assessment is made at one and five minutes after birth, and a baby with a score of at least 5 at one minute, or at least 8 at five minutes, seldom gives rise to any concern.

During the first 24 hours your baby will have a full examination by the doctor, who will check every detail. At this time less obvious problems are identified, such as an unstable ('clicking') hip, minor degrees of cleft palate, undescended testicle, etc. If any treatment is required, arrangements can be made for this at once.

The brand-new baby

The newborn baby has a strong sucking reflex and if you are going to breastfeed, it is advantageous to put your baby to the breast as soon as practicable after the birth, while the sucking response is strong. The baby has a 'rooting' reflex which means that when touched on the cheek by the breast, he will turn his head instinctively towards the touch.

The newborn baby will grasp tightly an object placed in his palm or curl his toes when touched on the sole. The 'walking reflex' which makes him lift his feet alternately if held just standing on a table is very strong in the first days, gradually diminishing in the first few weeks.

He will respond sharply to a sudden noise, but will be soothed by a gentle rhythmic sound. The baby will respond to voices directly in front of him.

The baby can distinguish the outline of something in front of him. He can focus at about nine inches but will not hold the gaze for more than a few seconds.

The first month

Your baby may smile from the first few days but the responsive smile tends to appear from four weeks onwards.

Sleeping patterns differ widely; one baby will sleep much in the day, waking only to be fed and changed, while another will sleep very little, perhaps only a few hours. It is important to play with your baby, talk to him and cuddle him when he is awake. Babies carried close to their mothers, especially in chest-to-chest contact, often seem more contented than babies who are left alone.

At some times the baby may wave his arms and legs happily, but will do this more strongly when unwrapped and placed on a cold surface, often crying unhappily. You may notice this when he is placed on a cold plastic changing mat or in the cold scales at the baby clinic.

When lain on his tummy, he can turn his head from side to side, and when held against your shoulder he may hold his head clear of your shoulder for a moment. His hands are curled with the thumb inwards. During this month he will uncurl from the foetal position.

Two to three months

His hands are now open and he will start to discover his hands and feet. He will be delighted to discover the relation between grasping the beads across the pram and hearing the rattling noise they make. He will kick his legs in the air. He will be able to grasp an object when given it and will grab at your hair or beads or glasses.

When lying on his tummy he will raise his head and shoulders up from the mattress. He can now roll from his side on to his back.

He will look long and hard at things around him, especially his mother's face. He will respond more positively to speech, becoming quiet or kicking and gurgling happily. Now he really enjoys a time of play on the rug or a large bed. Talk to him and sing and give him the opportunity to 'talk back'.

Three to six months

Now he may be able to roll over from front to back. He will enjoy taking the weight on his feet and being bounced gently.

He will begin to sit up supported and will look around with great interest. When placed on his front, he will raise his whole chest from the floor or mattress and hold this position. He may now begin to draw his knees up under his body and rock.

He tries to work out how to grasp his feet and is delighted when he succeeds. He will reach out for objects and grasp them firmly. Now he needs to be allowed to work out how to reach objects and you should not place them in his hand. He only copes with one object at a time. He will accept strangers happily, especially if you are present.

Six months to a year

Your baby will now be able to sit up unsupported. He will probably be crawling, though some babies never crawl but shuffle along on their bottoms, sometimes with one leg tucked underneath; they usually start later than crawlers and also walk later, perhaps not until 18 months.

During this period he will start to pull himself on to his feet and then move around holding on to the furniture, stepping sideways. He will stand up with support or alone, and by one year many babies will take their first steps alone.

He now enjoys toys which make a noise (squeak or hoot, for instance), and will be happy banging a spoon on a saucepan or putting objects into containers. He has learned to release his grasp as the grasp reflex disappears, so he throws his toys away and will give objects to you.

He will watch animals and machines with interest. He recognizes members of the family and well-known friends approaching from 20 feet or more away. He will know his own name and turn when he hears it.

He can understand most of what is said relating to his daily life and he babbles loudly, tunefully and incessantly. He can repeat syllables in long strings.

He imitates adults' sounds and actions, such as 'pat-a-cake' and waving 'bye-bye', and enjoys playing 'peep-bo'.

He can drink from a cup and will try to feed himself with a spoon. He is now chewing his food.

He clearly distinguishes strangers from family, and may hide his face and cling to you when a stranger approaches.

The health visitor

When the baby is about a fortnight old, your health visitor will call. She is a nurse who has had special training in the care and development of babies and her first job is to answer your questions – any questions, about anything. To do with feeding perhaps, or when to pick the baby up, how much to play with him, why his motions have changed colour, where to get supplementary benefit, what the doctor meant about clicking hips, etc. She works closely with your GP and they will often collaborate on any problem you or your baby may have. The health visitor runs the clinic where you take the baby for medical check-ups and immunizations, and will keep in touch with you until your child is five years old.

Going to the clinic

In every area there are clinics to which you can take your baby for regular checks and immunizations. Because it is also a good opportunity to meet other mothers, your visit to the clinic may become a pleasant social event! Arrangements vary a little, but your health visitor will give you all the local details.

At the clinic, the baby will be weighed and you can see the progress in his growth. Of course, some babies are bigger than others, but there is a 'range of normal', and special charts have been designed which outline this range – separate ones for boys and girls, who differ in growth rate from a surprisingly early age. You will see that the chart also shows the normal rate of growth for a baby. This is a very important factor. After a few visits you will be able to check that your baby is growing at a normal rate.

Examinations will be carried out to check that the baby is developing and that he is able to do the things expected of a child of his age. Again, there is a range of normal and the tests will show if the baby is within this range. The ages at which tests for these developmental changes are done may differ from one area to the next, but are usually at about two months and eight months, when the hearing is also tested.

Your baby as an individual

All the talk about normal will not make you think that your baby is just like all the others – and of course he is not. From the moment he is conceived he is an individual in his own right and you will have the joy of watching him develop a personality and physique which are unique. The summaries above of what to expect will help you to look for particular features in his development; as each new one appears, take every opportunity to encourage him to exercise it. Treat him like a real person, not a toy, so that he can respond to you; and, above all, enjoy him! Never underestimate your own special, intimate knowledge of your own baby: you will know his patterns and reactions, likes and dislikes, fears and pleasures, sooner than anyone else.

Breastfeeding

Breastfeeding means giving your baby the nourishment which is most suitable for his digestive abilities. You are also making the closest contact possible, once the umbilical cord is cut. It is wise to prepare while you are pregnant (see pp. 55–8) and to learn as much as possible about it beforehand. There is much information about breastfeeding problems in this section. Don't be put off by this. You might experience one or two of them, but many women have no significant problems at all.

The early days

After delivery   When your baby is born the midwife will clear his airways of mucus so he can breathe and suck freely. He has the ability to suck before birth, so if you put him to the breast when he is given to you after delivery you will find that he will nuzzle around and look for food while this instinct is still very strong. The warmth of your body and the skin contact when you greet him is important communication.

The first few days   If you put your baby to the breast frequently in the first days of his life, he will receive the valuable colostrum, and his sucking will stimulate your breasts to produce milk in increasing amounts as his needs grow.

If extra fluids are advised in addition to breastfeeds, for example if your baby is jaundiced, they should be offered after the breast, and preferably by spoon or a teat with a small hole.

For relaxed and enjoyable feedtimes, a comfortable position for you both is important. If you sit up to feed, have a good back support and an extra pillow under the baby (across your knees) as he will feel quite heavy held on one arm. But if you have had stitches after an episiotomy, or a Caesarean, a reclining position can be more comfortable than sitting. Have your baby supported on the pillow and stroke the cheek nearest your breast with your finger. He will turn and open his mouth for food and comfort. The relaxation you learned in antenatal classes will be very useful at feedtimes: babies know if their mothers are tense and anxious. Concentrate on your baby, and let this be a time of special togetherness for you both.

Points to remember

To help your baby feed easily, hold him at the right height to reach the nipple. Make sure his chin is touching the breast so that the nipple goes well into his mouth. As he nuzzles and opens his mouth wide, see that he takes the nipple and areola on top of his tongue. His gums should be well over the areola and not just on the nipple.

Allow him to suck at both breasts for *brief but frequent periods* in the first few days, starting each feed on alternate sides. Gradually increase the length of sucking time on each side. Breastfed babies often wake after two or three hours and need feeding again, as breastmilk is digested quite quickly. If your baby wakes during the night, feed him as it will help balance your supply and his demand.

It is usual to feed a baby from both breasts at each feed, starting on alternate sides. If the baby has a preferred side,

Usual position for breastfeeding

start him off on the less favoured side (i.e. when he is at his hungriest) for a few feeds. The quality of your milk is always excellent and cannot disagree with the baby, but the 'end milk' is richer, containing more fat than the first gush, so try to ensure that he empties one breast each time. If you forget which side to start on, fasten a small safety pin in your bra strap to remind you, moving it from one side to the other with each feed.

If your baby is restless at the breast, check that his nose is not blocked or buried in the breast.

To persuade the baby to release the nipple, break the suction by gently pressing his lower jaw or by easing his mouth open with your finger so that air goes in and relieves the vacuum.

Many breastfed babies never need burping. However, if your baby swallows much air during a feed you might like to try. You can cradle him against your shoulder with one hand supporting his back, rocking gently but avoiding vigorous back-patting which could make him vomit. Alternatively you can hold him in an almost upright 'sitting' position, supporting his head with your hand. The air should bubble up easily. If it does not come up within a few minutes, there is no point in persisting as either he has not swallowed enough air to need to bring any up, or it will pass out naturally while he is asleep.

To wake a sleepy feeder, unwrap him and encourage him to stretch his arms and legs. Try changing his nappy.

You will find feed times easier to manage as your breast hardness subsides and you get more used to the baby's strong sucking. He will want to suck for longer periods and by feeding him when he asks, your supply and his demand will soon be adjusted, provided extra bottles are not constantly offered. If you find you are experiencing difficulties such as engorgement, or breast or nipple tenderness, see p. 147.

New babies lose some weight in the first few days. During this time all their systems are becoming active, and they empty the bowel and bladder of waste from their growth period in the uterus. At first the bowel movements are dark and like tar in colour and consistency (meconium), but this gradually changes so that they look greenish and then yellow as the breast milk is digested. Breastfed babies' motions may be very profuse and frequent in the first few weeks, but this is not important provided the motions are yellow when passed.

The baby may have regained his birthweight before he leaves hospital, at about eight to ten days. If he is to be test-weighed this cannot be assessed over less than 48 hours, as he will not take exactly the same amount at each meal – any more than you do!

Be patient and persevere. It can take several weeks for breast-feeding to become well-established.

When you get home

Tiredness   It is exciting to arrive home with a new baby, but you may also feel more tired than you anticipated. Tiredness is one of the greatest problems for any new mother, whether or

not she is breastfeeding, so be sure to sit or recline comfortabl
and to relax your face, shoulders and limbs as you start to fee
the baby. While your baby wakes you at night for feeds, a day
time rest is essential. Use your baby's longest sleeping period t
rest, rather than catch up on housework, and try to make life a
simple as possible for the whole family.

It is usually more expedient, and better for the milk supply, t
feed a hungry baby on demand for the first few weeks rathe
than try to make him wait.

If you lose confidence or get in a muddle, contact your NC
breastfeeding counsellor, or talk to someone who has fec
happily for longer than you have. Keep in touch with a helpfu
nurse, health visitor or friend, but avoid – for a while – anyon
who is discouraging about breastfeeding. Do keep going. Thi
is just a phase which will pass in a few days.

Diet and rest   It is important to eat well and drink enough
fluids (see the section on diet during lactation). Eat simple
nourishing meals and have a drink and a snack during the baby'
feedtimes as well as your usual tea breaks. Be sure not to ski
breakfast or lunch. This extra food will not cause you to put or
weight, but will provide the extra energy and calories that yo
need to feed a baby.

A few foods eaten by you may affect your baby and perhap
make him restless, give him colic or diarrhoea. These wi
probably be foods which you only eat occasionally, or to excess
Most laxatives will also have this effect. Smoking and stron
black coffee should be avoided as both nicotine and caffeine
pass through to the milk. One greenish bowel motion passed b
your baby is not important. If he passes several you shoulc
consult your doctor, in case the baby has an infection.

Your milk   When your baby cries you will probably feel the
let-down reflex: there is a tingling in your breasts and your milk
begins to flow in readiness for a feed. This is an exciting, proud
feeling for many mothers. The sensations can be quite strong
however, and if you want to ease them, press the heel of you
hand over the nipple area until it ceases. (If you are in public

you can do this unobtrusively by folding your arms.) Disposable breast pads, disposable nappy liners or nappy roll can be used inside your bra to absorb leakage, but do not allow them to become soggy or this will make your nipples sore. Men's handkerchiefs, old and soft from many launderings, can also be used; they are easily washed and dried for re-use.

Growth spurts   As your baby becomes more lively he may have considerable growth and appetite spurts. An extra feed in 24 hours, or demand feeding every two hours or so will stimulate your breasts to produce more milk. Supply should soon meet demand, usually after about 48 hours. Cuddle your baby and give him a little 'top-up' suckling if he seems tired but is reluctant to settle to sleep. Regular weighing will indicate how well he is thriving.

Pressures to wean   You will undoubtedly be subjected to some pressures to wean your baby early, but try to resist them. There are many advantages in continuing the breastfeeding for as long as you are both happy. Your baby can thrive on breast-milk alone until he is fully weaned to a cup, with no need for bottles. The ideal solution is to let your baby wean himself. He will give you very clear indications of tiring of the breast, any time from about six to 14 months or more. If you are seeking help to counteract adverse pressures, get in touch with your NCT breastfeeding counsellor, who can give you moral support. *To increase your supply, the golden rule is – feed your baby more frequently.* Short, frequent feeds help stimulate the production of more milk, so plan to feed your baby every two to three hours. You will need all the energy and rest you can get for this, so simplify your household tasks, be willing to accept practical help, and try to sleep when your baby sleeps during the day. Eat regular, nourishing meals and remember to eat or drink something during the baby's feedtimes as well, not because you should, but because it makes an easy reminder. You can also douche your breasts with alternate hot and cold flannels after a feed, to help stimulate their activity; do a little massage when drying them. Homoeopathic lac deflor may help, and taking vitamin B in the form of brewer's yeast may be useful, too.

Remember that babies cry for reasons other than hunger. If your baby has six or more wet nappies a day, normal soft yellow motions, and a steady weight gain, then he is getting enough milk. If he is still restless he may need the stimulation of your company and interesting things to see and do, rather than more food. Try carrying him round in a sling or papoose.

Weaning on to a bottle   If the baby is not gaining weight, if you are returning to work, or if you are not enjoying breast-feeding for any reason, you may need to wean him on to a bottle. Think about this carefully, but if you do decide to change to bottle-feeding, consult your health visitor for a suitable formula. To wean the baby, start by dropping one breastfeed completely in the middle of the day and substitute a bottle. After a few days, if your breasts are not uncomfortable, drop another feed. Continue until all the breastfeeds have been replaced by bottle feeds; this should take between two and four weeks. (It takes this long because the breasts reduce the amount of milk they are making only gradually.) If you were reluctant to give up breastfeeding but had to because the baby was not thriving, there is no reason why you should not go on putting him to the breast for as long as you both want to, in addition to his bottle feeds. If you have to return to work, it is possible to combine breast-and bottle-feeding.

Possible problems

Inverted or flat nipples   If this condition has been diagnosed during pregnancy you will probably have been wearing Wool-wich Shells to draw out your nipples. After your baby is born the use of an electric pump may help to pull them out, but the best treatment for inverted nipples is the vigorous sucking of your baby. You may need particular patience in the early days, especially if you become engorged (see below). Try to persevere, as the condition will improve.

The Natural Nursing Nipple Shield (available from the NCT) is often very helpful. It is made of rubber and is applied directly over the nipples. If you need to wear a shield for more than a few feeds, increase the baby's sucking time so that your nipples get sufficient stimulation to maintain the milk supply.

Sore nipples   Some tenderness at first is usual, particularly if you have a fair skin. To help prevent sore nipples, you should keep them supple and 'waterproofed' by applying lanolin or nipple cream after each feed. Dry them carefully after each feed and, if milk leaks between feeds, make sure that your nipples do not remain constantly damp. However, there are a number of things you can do if your nipples do become really sore.

Before feeding, relax, then hand-express a little milk from each breast to soften the areola so that the baby can take your nipple fully into his mouth. Start feeding from the less sore side first, as sucking is most vigorous at the beginning of a feed. When the first strong sucking has subsided, change to the sore breast and empty it, and then return to the first side. Remove the baby from the breast carefully by gently breaking the suction by pressing on his jaw. Dry your nipples thoroughly and use a healing cream, such as pure lanolin, after feeding. Avoid drying agents such as alcohol on the sore area.

Exposure to air helps natural healing: think how quickly the skin of a cut finger heals up when you remove the sticking plaster. So expose your nipples to the air while in the house or garden, or to the warm air of a hair-dryer or convector heater. Nylon tea strainers with the handles removed, worn inside your bra, help keep the air circulating around sore nipples (even if this idea does seem laughable!) However, make sure that they do not press into the breast tissue as this could cause blocked ducts (see below).

Sit one foot away from a light bulb and expose your nipples to the light for a few minutes at a time. If you have a sun-lamp, you can use it, but only very carefully – for *half a minute* the first day increasing by half a minute a day to a *maximum* of three minutes. Sunburnt breasts are extremely painful, so avoid them at all costs!

The Natural Nursing Nipple Shield, described above, will help protect the nipples while feeding. If necessary, you may take aspirin or paracetamol half an hour before feeding, if the pain is bad.

Engorgement   When the breasts first fill with milk they may become very tense and hard, with perhaps some swelling of the areola. This engorgement happens between the second and fifth day after delivery. It is not entirely due to the presence of milk; the milk-producing cells themselves enlarge under the stimulus of hormones, and the blood supply to the breasts is greatly increased. This initial engorgement, which may be quite painful, is only temporary.

Short, frequent feeds (if your hospital will allow it) will help reduce engorgement. Apply cold compresses or ice packs between feeds for comfort and to reduce the swelling.

You may need to express a little before you put the baby to the breast so that he can grasp the nipple correctly. Warm douching, or the application of a warm flannel, before a feed will help start the milk flowing.

Wear a good, supporting bra, as your breasts will be temporarily several inches bigger. The NCT's Mava Bra is designed with lacing at the back so it expands to fit comfortably at this time.

Do not offer the baby complementary feeds if you can avoid it as he will then be less hungry when he comes to feed from you and will not empty the breasts so efficiently. Avoid also too much expressing, as excess stimulation will increase the problem, unless your breasts become very lumpy, or your doctor or midwife advises it. The trick is to let the baby empty the breasts regularly but not to stimulate the supply further by any more expressing.

Cracked nipples   These occur when the skin of the nipples is actually broken rather than generally sore. Take the baby off the breast for 24 hours, or until the nipple has healed. Express the milk from the affected breast and feed it to your baby by spoon or bottle. Follow the treatment for sore nipples given above. When they feel better, restart feeding very slowly and examine your nipples after each feed. Check on the position in which you are holding the baby to make sure that he is not dragging on the nipples. Friar's Balsam mixed with lanolin may be put on the crack after feeds as a healing agent, but must be wiped off gently before the next feed. There is no need to wean your baby: with care the healing should be rapid.

Blocked ducts (see also section on 'Too much milk', p. 150). Sometimes your baby cannot quite keep pace with the supply, so one breast may not be adequately emptied. An ill-fitting or flap-fronted bra, or even the wearing of a bikini top, can cause blocked ducts. If you always sleep on the same side at night, a tender lumpy area may develop; or it may be caused by pressure from the baby's face or chin while feeding.

If you suspect a blocked duct, feed from that side first at each feed until the trouble clears, gently massaging with your fingertips towards the nipple, first below and then above the lumpy area, and apply gentle warmth so that the milk flows freely. Adjust the baby's position while feeding, if necessary, perhaps by tucking his body and legs under one arm. And try to lie on the other side at night.

Seek medical help if the trouble does not clear in 24 hours, or if you develop flu-like symptoms or have a raised temperature.

Mastitis   The symptoms of mastitis are a hard, reddened area in the breast after feeding, which is painful and warm to the touch, coupled with a shivery feeling and a temperature. This can be caused by milk stagnating in a breast which has not been sufficiently emptied, or by an infection entering the breast through a cracked nipple.

Take the antibiotics prescribed by your doctor, remembering that they may give your baby diarrhoea. Apply cold compresses, rest, and increase your fluid intake. Pay scrupulous attention to cleanliness, wearing a clean bra every day and changing breast pads frequently.

There is usually no need to stop breastfeeding. Stress when you see your doctor that you want to continue breastfeeding.

If mastitis is left untreated, an abcess may develop. Even then it is not normally necessary to stop breastfeeding. You can hand- or pump-express from the affected side, and continue to feed the baby from the good side until the abcess has drained.

Too much milk

Just as some women seem to be able to produce milk more readily than others, so there are others again who feel they produce too much. While it is gratifying to produce plenty of milk for one's baby, to be consistently overflowing with milk can be embarrassing for you and perhaps produce some problems for your young baby.

At feed time   There are several measures you can try to reduce the first flood of milk at feedtimes. Give your breasts a quick douche with cold water just before feeding; express a little milk at the beginning, before putting your baby to the breast; with your first and second fingers apply gentle pressure to the areola area to restrict the flow.

Take the baby off the breast after the first gush, which may have overwhelmed him. Give him time to get his breath back and to bring up any wind he may have gulped down. He may need to be held up against you and soothed with rocking and the contact of his head with your face. Calmer, quieter sucking may then follow.

Alternatively you can position yourself and the baby so that he sucks 'up-hill', either by holding him on a pillow above the level of the nipple, or by lying on your back while he lies across your body on his tummy, his head supported with the heel of your hand to prevent him burying his nose while sucking. Position an older baby so he is sitting up to feed.

Leaking   If your breasts leak between feeds, before feeds, or during the night, keep your bra comfortably firm and well-padded with a piece of nappy liner, breast pads, or folded men's handkerchiefs. To keep your skin as dry as possible, use pieces of one-way nappy liner next to the skin, but change the padding and lining frequently. For special occasions, a piece of water-proof fabric may be put between the padding and your bra or clothing, but if used too often or for too long this may make damp skin worse and more prone to soreness.

Wear loose and perhaps dark or patterned outer clothing, and at night put a thick towel or rubber sheet between the under-sheet and mattress. If you feel your milk begin to let down, press the heels of your hands firmly on the nipple and areola area until the tingling ceases.

A small amount of intitial let-down from one breast while feeding from the other may be absorbed by using a bra pad and keeping your bra fastened on one side while feeding. A larger amount may be caught in a Woolwich Shell or in a small bowl or coffee cup. Special care baby units are often glad to receive even an ounce of breast milk, so contact your local hospital, health visitor, or breastfeeding counsellor for information.

For babies already on a mixed diet, surplus breast milk can be mixed with solid food. It can be kept in a covered sterile container for up to three days in the fridge or six months in the freezer.

Your breasts may leak while making love; this may be lessened by having intercourse after a feed. Anxiety may also cause leaking, so talking over any problems with a breast-feeding counsellor or other sympathetic person may help.

Expressing   You should be careful not to express more than just enough to keep you comfortable and the ducts clear (see p. 152), as the overstimulation of too frequent expressing may perpetuate the problem.

Reducing the milk supply   If expressing excess milk for one or two feeds has not enabled the baby to catch up with your supply, try to reduce the amount of sucking in 24 hours. Be quite sure that the baby's crying really indicates hunger each time rather than boredom, wind, or some other discomfort. Excessive weight gain would indicate the baby's ability to manage with fewer or shorter feeds. If the baby is unhappy, try giving him a dummy to satisfy his need to suck. A pram ride or a change of scene may distract him and help him adjust to the new regime.

If you produce a lot of milk overnight, but are perhaps a bit short in the evening, collect the excess in the morning to top up with at tea-time, or wake the baby at night for an extra feed to relieve the pressure. Check that your diet is properly balanced and make sure that you are eating well at breakfast and lunch-time.

Experiment with reducing the amount you drink, but do not cut down drastically.

The baby's difficulties   The first gush of milk after the let-down and the fast flow can be rather overwhelming for even a hungry baby, especially if he is still small. He may gulp air as he tries to cope with the flow, and this can cause wind. Discomfort from the wind gulped down will need relief. Hold your baby against your chest, or lay him flat on his tummy. If he does not like this position, try raising the end of his mattress with a folded towel underneath (so that the wind can bubble out while he is asleep), or putting a warm towel on his tummy.

If he takes more milk than his digestive system can stand, he may also have a distended stomach, so his crying may be caused by discomfort rather than hunger. If he can digest the milk, he may become overweight; but breastfed babies usually regulate their intake and, even when they gain rapidly in the first few months, gain more slowly later. If overloading his stomach causes vomiting or frequent motions, he may not absorb enough milk and could become too thin and underweight. This may also happen if the baby takes a lot of fore-milk and little or none of the richer end-milk.

How to express and store breast milk

There is no need to express milk in the ordinary course of breastfeeding, but you may want to collect and store it in special circumstances: if your baby is in hospital or cannot suck and you want to collect all your milk to be given to him by bottle or tube; if you are going to be away from your baby temporarily and want to save up milk for one or more bottles while you are away; if you are breastfeeding your baby and also want to donate milk to a milk bank for premature and sick babies; if your doctor or midwife advises it; to relieve overfilling so that the baby can get a better grip on the nipple; if your nipples are cracked and you have to rest them.

The milk collects in 15–20 small reservoirs deep behind the areola and can be squeezed out through openings in the nipples. You may have done this on a small scale to express colostrum when you were pregnant. The method of milk collection you choose, and how often you do it, will depend upon your particular circumstances.

Methods of collection The simplest method, if you are feeding your own baby, is to catch drips from the other breast, in a sterile container, while the baby feeds. The baby does all the work and some mothers produce quite large amounts this way, especially in the early weeks.

Breast pumps work by applying a rhythmical suction to the nipple and the areola. They are efficient at extracting the milk and help to improve the shape of flat nipples.

The simplest form of breast pump is a hand-pump, which can be bought from some chemists. It is made of glass with a rubber squeeze bulb, and looks rather like an old-fashioned car horn. The glass has a flanged hole into which the nipple goes, at the other end it connects to the rubber bulb, and at the bottom is a reservoir for milk, holding up to 60 ml (2 fl oz). Squeeze as gently as possible until you get used to the action.

Electric pumps can be hired for home use in many areas and many maternity units have them. Their action is carefully designed to avoid damage to the nipple. In the majority of cases the electric pump is used by mothers of premature or ill babies who require nursing in special care baby units (see p. 177). Other uses are: relieving engorgement; increasing the milk supply; correcting inverted nipples; emptying the breast when a nipple is sore or cracked (though there have been cases where pump use has re-opened cracks); re-establishing a milk supply after giving up breastfeeding; maintaining a supply when the mother and baby are separated.

A number of NCT branches throughout the country have electric breast pumps for hire: instructions for use are provided.

How to express by hand   Hand-expressing is a means of emptying the milk from your breasts by using your hands to squeeze out the milk. It requires no special equipment, and some women find it very simple. Not everyone finds it easy to acquire the knack, and it is not very efficient at emptying the breast, so it is probably most useful if you have to express only a small amount for a short period.

The following instructions assume that you will express the left breast with the right hand, and vice versa, which many women find easy.

Wash your hands thoroughly. Lean forward and let your breast hang down. Stroke the breast very gently towards the nipple with a delicate finger-tip touch before and while you are expressing, to encourage milk to flow down the ducts. Support the left breast in the left hand and, with the right hand, squeeze the milk reservoirs by placing the tips of the thumb and first (or middle) finger on opposite sides of the areola, just on the outer edge.

Press the thumb and finger into the breast towards your rib cage, then squeeze them rhythmically together. The pressure must be very firm to get the first few drops of milk. The fingers must not slide over the skin of the areola or touch the nipple, but squeeze in behind the nipple.

Move the finger and thumb around to the other sides of the areola to make sure that all the reservoirs are emptied. Change hands (and breasts) frequently, to avoid tiredness.

When to express   If you are expressing all your milk for your own baby, you will need to express four or more times a day in order to maintain the milk supply. If you need to increase the supply, try expressing six times a day and use a pump.

CAUTION   It is not very often necessary to express milk during the normal course of breastfeeding, and too much expressing for no good reason may be damaging if not done properly.

Bottle-feeding

Bottle-feeding is an alternative to breastfeeding, when breast-feeding is not possible through illness, lack of help, choice, or the few medical conditions which contra-indicate breast-feeding. It is used occasionally to complement breastfeeding.

The aims are the same, whatever method of feeding is used: to promote the bond between mother and baby, and to provide the best available nutrition. With any new baby, the senses of hearing, touch, and smell are more developed than sight, so that skin contact and warmth play a part in feeding, as does talking to the baby. Feeding time is a special time in which to learn to know and love each other.

Bottle-feeding has been known through the ages, but it is only in the last fifty years that it has become safe enough to be widely used. In the last five years, further safety measures have been introduced in this country.

Bottle-feeding generally means using cows' milk or a modification of cows' milk. Soya bean substitutes can be prescribed for babies who have an allergy to cows' milk, and modified goats' milk is also used occasionally.

Milk is a complete food, a fluid containing protein, sugar, salts, fats, and some vitamins, and each species of mammal provides a milk which is uniquely suited to its own young. To adapt cows' milk for human babies, careful scientific modification is necessary to bring it closer to human milk, although there are still many differences.

Instructions for preparing feeds vary with each manufacturer and are clearly indicated on each packet. These must be followed carefully, if a safe and correct formula is to be achieved.

Bottle-feeding is more cumbersome than breastfeeding, but it is not necessarily more difficult and can be carried out as tenderly, providing much pleasure for the baby.

Points to remember

Adequate sterilization is vital: cold-water sterilization of all equipment using a hypochlorite solution (e.g. Milton) is simple and generally preferable, but boiling for a minimum of ten minutes can be equally effective.

A modified milk suitable for infants under six months should be chosen for your new baby. Check with the midwife or health visitor for a suitable brand.

Prepare each feed as instructed, using only the measuring scoop provided. *Do not* overfill the scoop, compress the powder in it, or add additional scoops.

Do not store prepared feeds, except covered in a refrigerator, and then for no longer than 24 hours. If travelling, do not carry warm feeds, for instance, in thermos flasks, because bacteria multiply rapidly in warm milk. Keep it cold and then warm it immediately before feeding.

Modern modified milks are safer than the older brands in common use until quite recently, but do not always satisfy a baby for the 'routine' four hours. The pattern is more like breastfeeding, with varying amounts of feed being taken and at varying intervals.

Remember that babies are often thirsty and not always hungry. Offer extra water or add 15–30 ml ($\frac{1}{2}$–1 fl oz) of extra water to the feed. Your baby may not be able to cope with the manufacturer's recommended strength of feed and if he possets a lot (brings back small quantities of milk after feeds), the feed can be made weaker by adding 30 ml (1 fl oz) of extra water *or* by omitting one scoop of the formula.

Modified milks contain essential vitamins. Extra vitamins are unnecessary and extra vitamins A and D can be harmful.

Feeds may be given cold, warm or at room temperature, but

must never be given hot. Test the milk by running a few drops on the inside of your wrist. It should feel neither warm nor cold. A bottle should not be re-heated, and left-over formula should be thrown away.

There are variations in shapes of teats and in sizes of holes. A medium-holed teat is the usual choice, but continual sterilization does alter the size of the hole. Check daily, especially if the baby tires easily during feeding.

It is usual for young babies to swallow air when feeding and it is advisable to stop once or twice to allow the baby to burp. This can be achieved by sitting the baby up and gently rocking him or rubbing his back. The teat needs to be released frequently to let air enter the bottle.

Clean the bottles with a bottle-brush – first with cold water, immediately after feeding, to remove the protein film – then with hot soapy water to remove the fat. Rub the teats with salt, inside and out. Return everything to the chemical sterilizing solution, which should be made up daily.

Remember to talk to and cuddle your baby during feeding times and never leave him alone with a bottle, even for a moment, in case he chokes.

You must continue to sterilize your baby's bottles for as long as milk is offered in them.

Early days

Your baby may be sleepy at times at first. This will improve as he gets older. Bowel movements alter in the early days, and bottle-fed babies are sometimes slightly constipated. Extra water helps, but if it is a problem, ask your health visitor for advice.

New babies need time and energy spent on them, and you may well be tired. Eat sensibly and rest when you can; you will feel better for it.

Introducing solid foods

During the first four months, a diet of milk and, in some cases, a vitamin supplement, is all that is required to ensure an alert and contented baby with a healthy weight gain of 113–200 g (4–7 oz) per week, which should taper off to about 450 g (1 lb) a month by the seventh month. After the fourth month, little tastes of puréed foods can be offered in order to pave the way for a more varied diet at approximately six months.

If your baby is over four months old, and despite more frequent milk feeds, seems interested in more, this will probably mean readiness for solid food. If you are breastfeeding, you judge by the baby's demands; if you are bottle-feeding, the baby may be taking 1 litre (30–35 fl oz) of milk a day when he starts to want solids.

Start with very small quantities – about a teaspoonful – and do not make a great fuss about the procedure. It does not matter, from a nutritional point of view, if the baby does not eat the food. Do not interpret any rejection of the food as a rejection of you.

Starting mixed feeding

Usually the 2 p.m. or lunchtime feed is a good one at which to start solids. If you are breastfeeding, offer the breast before the solids to maintain your milk supply. Later, one breast can be offered, then the solids, and then the other breast. This ensures that at least one breast is emptied at each feed. If you are bottle-feeding, start by giving most of the milk first, then the solid food, slowly decreasing the amount of milk offered as the amount of solid food is increased. As your baby becomes more interested in solid foods, he may prefer them first and his milk at the end of the meal.

Vegetables and fruit make a better introduction than cereal. At first purée or sieve the food to a smooth, semi-liquid consistency. A manual food blender is best for small amounts: larger amounts can be prepared in an electric blender if you have one. Your baby will suck at the spoon to begin with and perhaps spit the spoonful out simply because he is not used to dealing with food in this form, but he should soon acquire the new skill. If he rejects it absolutely, leave it for a few days and try again. This may happen several times. Home-made purée will keep in the fridge for up to 48 hours.

Quantities

No more than one teaspoonful should be offered the first time. Increase amounts very slowly so that after two to three months the baby is having a first course of protein (such as beans, cheese, meat, or fish) with vegetables and a second course of pudding or fruit – about 100–150 g (4–6 oz) in all – with a drink of juice or water afterwards. If the baby is uncomfortable, colicky, or has unusual bowel motions, you are probably going too fast. When one food is accepted, add another, gradually increasing the variety. Babies can take time to get used to savoury foods, so concentrate on bland vegetables such as carrot, potatoes, and cauliflower first.

Do's

In a family with a history of allergies, consult your doctor about which foods to delay introducing, usually eggs, wheat, and cows' milk.

Introduce each new food individually, so that foods which disagree with the baby may be readily identified. Sieve or purée foods very carefully in the beginning, progressing to mashing with a fork at about six or seven months. Offer juice or water by cup at about five months; try again a week later if it is rejected.

As soon as your baby can hold a spoon, offer him one while you are feeding him and encourage him to scoop up some of his own dinner. Guide his hand to get the food into his mouth. Do not be dismayed if he throws it on the floor; put a plastic sheet or cloth under the high chair.

Include the baby in family meals at least once a day when

solids have been established, to encourage the child's enjoy-
ment of his food and imitation of others at the table.

When your baby is having a full lunch or dinner of first and
second courses, offer diluted fruit juice (not squash) or plain
boiled water afterwards instead of the breast or bottle feed.

If the baby is ready, start small amounts of solid food at
breakfast or tea when he is six or seven months old. If you progress at this rate, he will probably be having three meals a day,
mainly from the family menu, by nine to twelve months of age.
Continue with milk at breakfast and tea, also at bedtime if
required. All babies will differ, so this should only be a general
guide.

Don'ts

Do not offer new solids to a baby crying with hunger; this will
annoy him and colour his opinion of solid food. Do not transmit
your own likes and dislikes. Your voice, tone, and facial expressions tell all!

Never re-use a tin or jar of food into which you have dipped
the eating spoon. The saliva on the spoon will start a breakdown
of the food causing it to decay rapidly. Do not reheat food left
over from the baby's meal.

Avoid the use of sweets. Remember that a 'sweet tooth' is
developed, not inherited, and do not automatically sweeten
foods. Babies over a year old can have raisins instead of sweets.
Most fruits, drinks, and cereals are tolerated without sugar.

Do not add salt to a baby's food.

If you are bottle-feeding, do not add cereal to the milk as this
prevents the calcium in the milk being used effectively.

Do not leave a young baby of six months alone with food on
which he may choke or gag.

First foods

Fruits are ideal beginners. Puréed and sieved apples, pears, and
peaches, and ripe mashed banana, can be prepared in amounts
to last several days and stored in a clean container in the fridge.

or freezer in covered plastic ice-cube trays. When the baby can chew (around six to eight months), he can be given very thinly sliced raw apple or pear to hold and chew.

Vegetables   Virtually any puréed vegetables can be served. Skinned, puréed tomato is particularly convenient. After the first year, well-washed and scrubbed vegetables can be given raw, e.g. carrot sticks.

The best way to cook fruits and vegetables is to put just enough water into a saucepan to cover the bottom. While the water is boiling, drop in the finely chopped fruit or vegetables, bring back to the boil rapidly and reduce the heat to simmer. Cook for the minimum time possible; do not add salt to the vegetables.

Meats   These foods are fibrous and so must be cooked very well and blended thoroughly. Add some of the meat juices, broth, or water to moisten. Use any lean meat that you eat; liver and kidneys are especially suitable as they contain lots of iron. Avoid meat which has been ground by the butcher as the surfaces have been handled and they are usually high in fat and fibre content. You can, of course, mince your own meat. At eight to ten months, meat can be offered minced and the baby can chew on a defatted and meaty cooked bone which has no sharp edges or splinters. Crisp bacon at this time is a good finger food (i.e. food which babies can hold in their fingers).

Fish   White fish may be introduced cautiously after six months, but leave oily fish such as sardines, herrings, or mackerel until the second year, and do not give a baby salted or smoked fish such as kippers or smoked haddock. When it is fully cooked the fish will separate easily into flakes; if cooking fillets or cutlets a white curd-like substance will form between the flakes indicating that the fish is cooked. Be careful to remove all bones.

Vegetarian food   Instead of meat and fish, vegetarians can offer 'soya meats' (those which do not contain monosodium glutamate), lentil and nut roasts and mixed vegetable proteins suitably puréed. (Suggestions for vegetarian menus can be had from The Vegetarian Society, 55 Marloes Road, London W5.)

Eggs   After six months, begin using the yolk only, raw or cooked, sieved and stirred into fruit or vegetable purées. Do not introduce the white of the egg until you are sure that the yolk is tolerated.

Cheese   Any mild, finely grated hard cheese can be given, perhaps added to a white sauce and cooked to a smooth paste. Cottage and cream cheese can also be sieved with the baby's food. Melted cheese should not be given to a baby as it becomes stringy and indigestible.

Breads and cereals   Cereals should never be the predominant part of a meal. Introduce rice, oats or barley cereal first and delay the use of wheat cereal as some babies may be allergic to the gluten in wheat flour. At about seven months, toasted bread or rusks are excellent finger foods and teething aids, but the baby needs to be watched while eating them to see that he doesn't choke.

Milk and milk puddings   Introduce small amounts of cows' milk after the sixth month, in a cup, at mealtimes. This should be scalded and diluted until the baby is one year old. Milk puddings, custards, or junkets can be served as a second course with fruit. Yoghurt too can be included if the baby likes it. Do not force cows' milk on your child if he does not like it.

Tins and jars of baby foods   These are useful for convenience (though expensive), but read the label carefully before buying. The contents are listed in order of their quantities, largest amounts first. Avoid those containing large amounts of cereal, wheat starch, or sugar.

A balanced diet

Adults and children should eat some foods containing each of the following daily: proteins, vitamins, carbohydrates/fats (see p. 36). Babies should not have very spicy foods, fruit squashes, unripe fruit, fruit with many seeds, coffee, cream cakes, and processed cereals. They may, however, be given very weak tea.

Points to remember

Mealtimes should be happy, so don't force food on your child. Reintroduce any rejected foods without fuss at a later time. Always be ready to mark time if the baby is teething or off colour. Be guided by the baby's reaction: if he is not forced he will soon regain his appetite. Don't equate food with love: when he rejects your cooking, he is not rejecting *you!*

A hungry baby will be eager and interested; if he just plays with the food and tries to throw it around, he is probably not hungry enough. Give him less next time.

Encourage independence: a child should be allowed to feed himself as soon as he wants to try. From seven to nine months provide part of each meal chopped or sliced so that he can finger-feed himself.

Things you will need

Getting a household ready for a first baby can seem to involve an incredible number of details and preparations for all kinds of possibilities. Advice will come from everywhere – from family and friends as well as from babycare manufacturers – so you will need to plan which of the many possible additions to your equipment you will want. If you know that people may be wanting to give you something for the baby, you may find that a list of possibilities is helpful.

The basics are:

A place to sleep

Carrycot, basket even a box or drawer with a suitable lining and mattress
(eventually a pram and/or cot)

Sheets

Blankets/pram or cot covers/shawls (especially washable ones)

Clothes and a place to keep them
Nappies and pins

Liners

Plastic pants

Babygrow suits or nightgowns

Vests

Cardigans

Outdoor clothing according to season (e.g. for winter – hats, bootees, top-to-toe suit with a hood and feet, mittens)

A place to feed which is comfortable for you

Laundering requisites
Buckets for used nappies to soak

Soaking/sterilizing solution

Soap or detergent, fabric conditioner

Nappy-changing requisites and a place to change – warm; comfortable for you both

Something to remove bowel motions from skin (e.g. cotton wool/toilet roll/wet flannel)

Nappy cream/vaseline/oil/powder/or lotion

Spare nappy pins

Bath requisites and place to bath – warm; comfortable for you both

Baby bath/washing up bowl/or kitchen sink

Baby soap and shampoo

Towels, flannels, sponge

(oil/cream, powder)

Basic care of your new baby

Mothering and fathering are a matter of common sense and individual taste. There are few right or wrong ways to do things, just as there is no standard way of being a daughter, wife, son, or husband. You and your baby will establish a way of life which suits you all best; the fact that your methods may drive someone else crazy is immaterial. There are no 'musts' about nappy changing, bathing, doing the laundry, or dressing the baby: be as unsystematic or meticulous as you like. The baby will know only whether or not you are happy and confident in your handling of him – and that is all he will care about.

If you have any problems they are likely to be caused by lack of experience, and only time can rectify that. People do not expect to be able to type the moment they sit down in front of a typewriter, or to be able to drive the first time they find themselves at the wheel of a car. It is the same with parenthood – it takes time and practice. If this is your first baby, you may find the following guidelines helpful, but make your own variations and discoveries. Ask your parents, friends, and health visitor for advice too, but feel free to pick and choose what suits you from the abundance of advice you will be given!

Clothing

Babies do not care how they look. They just want to be warm
and dry and they loathe being dressed and undressed. You will
probably not need many first-size clothes, just vests, babygrow
suits, or nightdresses and cardigans. As far as possible get things
that open either all at the back or all at the front so that you
need not turn the baby over more than once when dressing or
undressing him. Avoid long strings and ribbons; they soon get
sucked and chewed and can be dangerous. Mittens are best
made in fabric rather than knitted, so that there are no loose
loops in which little fingers can be caught, but both these and
bonnets are only necessary in cold weather. A couple of soft
shawls will envelop the baby snugly when carrying him from
room to room – again avoid long fringes or knitted patterns
with large holes. You can tell whether or not the baby is warm
enough by feeling the skin under the back of his collar.

Changing nappies

Nappies seem to preoccupy everyone in discussing babycare.
The point is to keep the baby reasonably clean and dry and not
to complicate the matter further. At first you may feel that it is
all rather messy and unpleasant, but eventually even the most
squeamish of people find they can deal quickly and efficiently
with their own babies' excreta.

It is a false economy to skimp on the quality and quantity of
the towelling nappies you may buy. Thick nappies do not need
to be changed so frequently and should retain their absorbent
texture. You will need about $1\frac{1}{2}$ to $2\frac{1}{2}$ dozen depending on
your laundering and drying arrangements. At first, a new baby
can use about five or six nappies a day if he is changed after
most feeds.

There are three basic ways of putting on babies' towelling
nappies and the proponents of each method swear by it as 'the
only sensible way'! The three methods are illustrated below.
Try them out and see which one suits your baby best.

A. KITE SHAPE

1. Fold sides into centre as shown.
2. Fold top and bottom corners inwards, thus producing equal thickness everywhere.
3. Fold round baby's legs and pin at sides.

B. AMERICAN SHAPE

1. Fold nappy so that there are three thicknesses lengthwise (for a tiny baby fold into four so that the resulting strip is narrower).
2. Fold lower third up to make a thicker part to go at front or back, as required.
3. Simply fold round baby's legs and pin at sides.

C. ORIENTAL SHAPE

1. Fold nappy in half upwards.
2. Fold in half again, left to right.
3. Draw top layer of nappy from top right corner over to the left, holding other layers down, so that corner 'x' (see stage 2) arrives at top left centre (see stage 3).
4. Reverse whole nappy face downwards.
5. Fold straight edge on left into the centre, leaving the triangular 'wing' behind.
6. Fold thick strip between baby's legs and pin to 'wings'.

Plastic pants come in various types. Avoid those with very tight elastic around the legs; they can cut into the baby's flesh and make nappy rash worse by preventing the circulation of air around the nappy inside. Tie-on pants make a neat 'parcel' of the nappy and allow air circulation without any constriction at the top of the legs. Pants which fasten with poppers at the sides and have padded leg-holes are also comfortable for the baby and can be obtained in appropriate sizes. Some babies can never wear plastic pants because their skins are too delicate. Two towelling nappies make an adequate substitute. In any case, you may wish to avoid plastic pants as far as possible for a very young baby – imagine your own body steaming under a tight plastic mackintosh 24 hours a day, seven days a week!

Throw-away nappy liners are very useful for disposing of your baby's bowel motions and will help prevent staining of towelling nappies. Some of the more expensive disposable liners can be soaked, washed, and re-used, assuming they have only been wet, not soiled. One-way nappy liners are excellent for keeping your baby's bottom dry, but be careful not to clog the material with ointment or cream.

Have everything ready before you pick up the baby to change his nappy, so that you do not have to keep putting him down while you rush off to find something. It maddens him and will madden you.

If, for any reason, your baby develops nappy rash, expose his bottom to the air as much as possible (though this may involve lots of puddles, particularly with boys!) Try various proprietary ointments, vaseline, or ask your doctor or health visitor's advice about available brands. Skin varies so much between individuals that a cream which will work wonders for one baby may have no effect at all on his siblings.

If your baby is taking antibiotics (or you are taking them and breastfeeding him) do not use zinc and castor-oil cream on his bottom as this itself may cause a rash. Do not use it either if your baby has thrush.

The world will not cave in around your ears if the baby's

nappy is not changed at the middle-of-the-night feed. If he tends to produce a lot of urine which leaks into the cot over-night, try putting on two nappies: thick and thin towelling nappies, or a towelling nappy and a disposable one. A one-way nappy liner should ensure that the skin does not become sore.

The safest place for the baby to be when he is being changed is on the floor. He cannot fall anywhere!

Bathing

It is not necessary to bath a baby every day, so long as he is kept clean. Again, the matter can be made to seem unnecessarily complex. The main points to remember are: keep the baby warm; have everything ready in advance; wash his face and scalp first and his bottom later; and hold him firmly.

The usual way to bath a baby is in a special baby bath, but you can use a large washing-up bowl or a sink where the sharp taps have been covered by flannels. Before you bath the baby, wrap a large bath towel around your middle and have the room warm enough for you to bath him in a leisurely way. Check with your elbow or the inside of your wrist that the water is comfort-ably warm: babies don't like water too hot. Have everything ready to wash, dry and re-dress the baby before you undress him. Remember, you don't need much water, and as long as you wash his face and bottom the process need not be pro-longed. Hold him on your lap and wash his face, then use a tiny amount of baby shampoo to wash his head thoroughly. Hold his head over the bath to rinse away the suds. Handling a slippery small baby for a bath is an art and at first feels very precarious. Lower him gently into the water, with the back of his head resting against your left wrist and your left finger and thumb grasped firmly around his left arm just below the armpit, and your right hand under his legs or bottom. Until you are experienced at this, simply hold him there, just swishing the water gently around him with your right hand. If he shows any fright, try holding his arms firmly against his chest and he will be reassured. Lift him out and wrap him quickly in a warm towel, and let him feel secure and enveloped in comfort before you pat him dry, powder, and dress him.

It is not necessary to use soap or any other washing agent. The baby is not 'dirty' in the conventional sense of the word, so if you are worried about dropping him when he is slippery, just sponge him with the bath water.

The trickiest parts of a new baby to dry are the folds of skin under the arms and in the neck. Be careful, too, to dry in the groin and behind the ears. Avoid putting powder on wet patches; it just makes a 'pudding'.

There is no 'correct' time to bath a baby, the choice is yours. However it is not fair – on you or the baby – to give him a bath when he is very hungry, so do it between feeds when he is awake or, if it does not make him sick, after a feed. Some babies find baths very soothing and, if yours has a crying time, a warm luxurious bath may help to quiet him.

If your baby hates being bathed in the conventional way, you can try taking him into the ordinary bath with *you* (it may give you more confidence to have a non-slip mat on the bottom of the bath). Get in and out of the bath with the baby held firmly against your shoulder with one hand, and use the other to support yourself. Lie in the bath and sit him, or lie him, on your chest (or propped up, facing you, with his back supported against your raised thighs). Your presence and the reassuring nearness of your breasts should make the baby quite relaxed, and this mutual bathtime will be a happy and privately loving time for both of you. Keep the water comfortably warm but not too hot for the baby.

Laundry

A small baby generates an incredible amount of washing. Since the turnover is rapid, it is essential to see that everything is adequately aired. Ironing, incidentally, is not one of the essentials in the life of a new baby, or of a new mother, and can safely be omitted.

If washing by hand see that things are well rinsed, and whether by hand or machine, do not use too much detergent or soap powder. If you use nappy-sterilizing solution (or diluted house-hold bleach, or even washing soda) to soak nappies, they do not need boiling. Do not leave them in the solution too long, or it will smell revolting. Make up a fresh solution each day.

Sunshine will help to bleach nappies and rainwater softens them, so if you have enough it is a good idea to hang them out for a blow on the line whatever the weather. A tumbledrier is very useful for drying clothes and nappies or, if your home is centrally heated, the radiators will be useful too. White nappies hanging over white radiators do not look too obtrusive.

Fabric conditioner will help keep the nappies soft, but be sure to check that it does not cause an adverse reaction on your baby's skin. A compromise is to use the conditioner every two or three washes.

Socializing

Some mothers are most attracted to their babies when they are very tiny, seeing them as wonderful complex little people who somehow encompass the wisdom of the ages together with an awesome 'newness'. They find their maternal instincts are strongest when the baby is at his most dependent.

Others feel that very new babies do little but eat, sleep, and cry, and think that for the first month or so babies need atten-tion primarily for feeding, cleaning, and comforting. Some new parents feel that their very new babies are rather unrewarding companions: they seldom smile, their eyes wander, they don't reach out to people, they don't gurgle in recognition or even laugh when tickled. This is strictly true. However, what new babies can do is limited but can be endearing if you know where to look: any tiny baby will curl his hand around your finger if you touch his palm; many will visibly relax if you stroke their feet, or legs, or foreheads; some will push their feet against your hands if you do 'cycling' or 'knee-bending' exercises for them while they are lying down; they seem to fit almost miraculously into the crook of your arm or the curve of your tummy or the hollow of your neck and shoulder. If you put your hand on your baby's back or abdomen you can feel his stuttery, feathery breathing; if you put a (clean) finger into his mouth you can feel the power of his sucking reflex; if you watch him sleeping, or sometimes if you sing or talk while he is asleep you can see him making the same wriggling movements which he made before he was born.

Appreciating a tiny baby means understanding that he is in the first month or so making tremendous adjustments, and then watching for the responses he can make. His repertoire will expand, and will move from the instinctive responses of the first weeks to the intentional interaction of the later.

Restless babies   Some babies are more excitable than others and some lead an energetic and extrovert social life almost from the start. If you have this sort of baby it is sensible to adapt your life to his and be prepared to take him around with you, in a sling or on an adjustable seat, as you work. As babies get older they like to have something to watch, but bear in mind that interesting sights are no substitute for interesting company. You may like to keep the baby in the room with you all day, whatever you are doing. There is no reason for him to be banished to a far-away bedroom, like an invalid, when he sleeps.

Babies all over the world are carried on their mother's bodies and the evidence seems to suggest that this keeps them snug and feeling secure. In the Western world, baby slings are becoming popular, both for ease of transport and to provide psychological comfort for restless babies. It is no reflection on you, however, if you have the sort of baby who loathes being handled and prefers a more solitary existence. If your baby cries constantly, you could try carrying him around in a sling during the day, as you do things around the house. This will not make him extra-dependent on you in later life, but will help give him a secure start, and he will soon feel confident enough to tackle independence. If your baby tends to bring up mouthfuls of stale-smelling milk when held upright in a sling, he (and your clothes!) might do better if you put him in a baby sling where he lies across your body instead. Encourage him to sleep between feeds, otherwise – as some recent research has suggested – his growth may be slowed.

Ailments

You will find many specialist books which discuss childhood ailments in detail. It is always difficult to gauge the seriousness of childhood ailments, especially with a first child and particularly in the middle of the night. You should not hesitate to contact your GP if you are really worried.

However, mothers with medical or paramedical backgrounds should guard against magnifying their children's ailments out of all proportion. When you are familiar with the symptoms of serious disease it is easy to imagine that your own baby's illnesses are more severe than they really are.

Practising

As prospective parents you may want to use visits to relatives and friends with babies or small children as discreet 'practice sessions', perhaps taking the children out for the afternoon or looking after the baby on your own for a time. Valuable though these 'dummy runs' may be, do not allow yourselves to be overwhelmed or put off by the children's behaviour. Your own family will arrive one at a time (usually!) and you will be the ones to decide their lifestyle.

The ill and premature baby

Some babies are born needing special care. There are many reasons – some of the more common ones are described below – but most mean that the baby will go to a 'special care baby unit' to ensure that he receives the extra medical attention he requires.

Keeping in touch

When the baby is in a special care unit both parents should visit as much as possible. Do not be intimidated by all the equipment, and do not feel that you will be in the way, no matter how often you visit. The nursing and medical staff are there to help you and your baby. If he is ill in the incubator reach in and hold his hand and comfort him. Talk to him so that he gets to know the sound of your voice. Once he is better you can take him out and give him a cuddle, and some units will let you give the tube feeds. Always ask the staff of the unit to explain what all the bits of apparatus do, since they will always appear somewhat strange and perhaps frightening to you when you first see them.

There is of course no reason why your special care baby should not benefit from your milk, in fact breast milk and colostrum are of particular value to him. From the start, learn to use a breast pump (see p. 177) to express your milk which can then be given to your own baby. If there is any surplus it can be used to benefit other babies. Once your baby weighs about 1·7 kg (3¾ lb) and is well, he will be transferred to a cot and when you come in you will be able to bathe and change him and establish him on breastfeeding. When the doctors judge that he is well enough, you will be able to take him home.

Small babies

Small-for-dates babies   These babies are mature but weigh less than normal for their length of gestation, and they can usually go with their mothers to the postnatal ward. However because they are small they have poor nutritional reserve which can cause the glucose level in their blood to become very low during the first 48 hours. If prolonged this can damage the brain and cause subsequent handicap. To detect it, the small-for-dates baby needs heel prick blood tests for glucose estimations three to four times a day during the first 48 hours. During this period he can go to the breast to get the benefit of colostrum, but since you will be producing very little milk he will need to have complementary bottle feeds to prevent his blood glucose getting too low. Occasionally (although rarely) this fails to keep the glucose level up and intravenous glucose will have to be given. Once lactation is established the baby can transfer to full breastfeeding.

Premature babies   Babies of less than 2 kg ($4\frac{1}{2}$ lb) birthweight or less than 34 weeks' gestation usually need to be admitted to a special care baby unit. It is important to remember that although your baby is in the special unit, he is an entirely healthy little human being, and only needs to be there because of his environmental and feeding requirements.

In the unit, many babies are in incubators to keep them warm, to facilitate giving extra oxygen if necessary, and to make it easier for the nurses to keep a close watch on them in case their condition alters. Many premature babies, due to their immaturity, breathe irregularly and may even stop breathing, although they are otherwise completely well. They are therefore routinely laid on an 'apnoea' mattress (apnoea means 'no breathing') which sounds an alarm if the baby stops breathing, thus calling the nurse to come and stimulate him to breathe again before any harm is done.

Most babies under 34 weeks' gestation cannot suck on a nipple (yours or a bottle's) and need to be fed every two to three hours through fine plastic tubes passed through their noses into their stomachs.

Sick premature babies   With good management most of these babies now survive without any long-term handicaps. Between 28 and 30 weeks (when the baby weighs about 1 to 1.5 kg ($2\frac{1}{4}$–$3\frac{1}{4}$ lb) he has an 80 per cent chance of surviving, and more than 19 in 20 babies of more than 30 weeks' gestation and 1.5 kg ($3\frac{1}{4}$ lb) birthweight will survive.

(a) Hyaline membrane disease, or respiratory disease syndrome (RDS)
These are two names for one disease which is very common in

premature babies. It develops within four hours of birth, and happens because the baby has immature lungs. There is no specific treatment and the baby has to be helped to get over the illness himself, especially by giving him extra oxygen. The disease lasts five to seven days, and once resolved leaves no after-effects.

During the illness frequent checks on the level of oxygen and various other chemicals in the baby's blood will be made by passing a fine plastic tube (catheter) into his bloodstream through his umbilicus. This does not hurt or disturb the baby, and is used for taking blood and for giving intravenous fluid or blood transfusions when necessary.

Around your baby's incubator will be various machines to record his heart-rate and respiration from electrodes fixed to his chest, to record the concentration of oxygen he is breathing, and infuse accurately small amounts of fluid through the umbilical catheter. The 10 per cent of these babies who have the worst lung disease will need a ventilator.

(b) Jaundice

Many babies develop jaundice. This rarely does any harm, but very high levels can cause brain damage. If there is a risk of this, the baby needs extra fluids (water or glucose) if your lactation is not fully established, though you can still put him to the breast. If this does not control the jaundice he will be placed naked under bright lights to bleach the yellow pigment out of his skin and blood (phototherapy). His eyes will be covered to protect them from the bright light.

(c) Other illnesses

Any illness, such as pneumonia or convulsions, can occur in a new baby, and will necessitate admission to the special care baby unit.

The malformed baby

One in about forty children is born with some malformation.

Many of these are satisfactorily corrected by an operation but about 15 per cent of the malformed babies die shortly after birth, with some condition that cannot be treated.

If your baby has a malformation the medical staff will come and talk with both of you if possible soon after the delivery to explain the situation. You will be bewildered and miserable, and very little of what is said the first time will make sense, so do not be afraid to ask to see them again so that all your questions may be answered.

With some malformations the baby will be ill and admitted to the special care baby unit. You should always go and visit him, even if the condition is very likely to be fatal. If it is not, an operation may correct all his problems, and like any other new-born child he needs his mother and father from the start. With many of these malformations you will be encouraged to look after your baby yourself, and he will be on the postnatal ward with you.

Establishing lactation using an electric breast pump

Use the pump according to the detailed instructions provided.
In the first three days after birth   Try to begin expressing within a few hours of birth, or certainly by the following day. Express at least five times a day, taking care to use the pump for a few minutes only on each side, increasing gradually over a period of several days (as would be the case for normal breastfeeding). Do not be concerned that the amount of colostrum you produce is small; this is quite normal.
Introducing the pump after the third day   Use of the pump may be delayed until the third day, or longer, according to your doctor's assessment of the baby's condition. By this time you may be experiencing some engorgement. The pump can help to relieve this. Introduce it gradually: three minutes each side, increasing to ten minutes each side. If your expressed breast milk is to be used, a longer period of expressing may be preferable, according to the comfort of your nipples. To increase the supply use the pump more often, and not for longer periods.

Establishing direct breastfeeding   At first the baby should spend minimal time at the breast to avoid giving you sore nipples, since the baby's sucking action is different from that of the pump. If your nipples do become sore (and this is quite common) follow the routine for prevention and treatment given earlier. In the first few days, if the baby is small or tires easily, it may be necessary to use the pump after feeds to maintain a good supply. Gradually increase the time the baby is at the breast. To encourage your baby to feed, express a little milk on to the nipple before putting him to the breast. Sometimes a baby will reject the breast because it feels unlike the bottle teat he is used to. Try a little honey or glycerine on the nipples for a few feeds only, or try using a nipple shield at the beginning of each feed. If you need the shield throughout the feed, try to nearly double the length of time at each breast to provide adequate stimulation of the milk supply. Decrease the use of the shield once feeding is well established. Demand feeding helps the transition to direct breastfeeding.

A baby transferring from bottle-feeding to breastfeeding may lose weight initially. This is normal, but do check regularly with your clinic. Once breastfeeding is established, your baby should gain weight steadily.

Remember that although things may seem hard at the initial stage of establishing breastfeeding with an ill or premature baby, the relaxed atmosphere of home will work wonders.

Sense of achievement   There is no doubt that the period of separation from your baby is one of great strain and anxiety, and maintaining lactation with a pump will help you through this time. It is not easy to 'feed' a pump at five o'clock in the morning, but when your baby is eventually established on the breast you will feel that the disruption to your life has been well worthwhile. If your expressed milk is being used to feed your own or other ill babies, you will experience a particular sense of achievement, but even if this is not possible the triumph of feeding your baby at home after a period of separation will be very satisfying.

Hygiene   Germs multiply rapidly in milk so it is important to avoid introducing any into it. Always wash your hands before collecting milk. Wash all utensils in hot soapy water to remove the milk film, and soak them in cold water if you cannot wash them immediately after use. For milk which is to be taken to hospital, the utensils should be sterilized by boiling for five minutes or by storing in an antibacterial solution like Milton. Do not put any metal objects in Milton.

Storage   Hospitals prefer glass containers and will supply pre-sterilized bottles, but if these are to be kept for several days before filling, it is a good idea to keep them in Milton.

Label each container with the date of collection of the milk and your name. If the container is in the ordinary part of the fridge you can top it up with more milk collected the same day.

The time you can store milk before it is given to the baby or treated (pasteurized or sterilized) in hospital depends on the temperature at which it is kept. Breast milk can be kept like cows' milk in the ordinary part of the fridge or can be deep frozen and kept up to six months. Any time spent at a higher temperature will reduce the total storage time, so chill the milk as quickly as possible. Stand it in cold running water if you do not have a fridge.

If you are taking milk to hospital every day and have no fridge, you can store it overnight in an insulated container with an ice-pack such as Freezella (from camping shops). The container can be made of polystyrene or cardboard with the bottom and sides lined thickly with newspaper, or a thickly padded bag. Leave as little air-space round the bottles as possible, and keep the ice-pack on top of them, covered by an insulated lid. Keep the container in the coolest, draughtiest place possible. You could ask the hospital to freeze one ice-pack for you while you are using another. This method is also useful if you have to leave milk out for collection, and when it is being transported.

Conditions for milk banks   Check with the hospital before you give milk to see what conditions they make. Some hospitals will not take milk which has been frozen, since they cannot be sure that the temperature has been constant. Report to the hospital if you have been in contact with any infectious disease.

Stillbirth

Whether a baby is stillborn or dies just after birth you will be numbed by what has happened. Why me? Why us? You will want to know the answers to many questions: Was it something we did? Will it happen again? Your obstetrician, paediatrician, and general practitioner will often be able to answer these questions for you and you may need to see them several times before you get a full grasp of what has happened. Remember that the paediatrician usually wants to do a postmortem on the baby. This may not only help him to prevent another baby dying of the same condition, but without it he may not be able to answer the question 'Will it happen again?'

If you know in advance that your baby will be stillborn, the staff will do their best to help you through the experience. You will probably discuss with them beforehand whether or not you and your husband will want to hold the baby when he is born. With this, as with other choices you will be given, you will be asked again later and can, of course, change your minds if you wish.

During the labour you and your husband will share unique parental grief and can start the process of mourning. Spare a thought for the midwife who will be sharing your feelings to a great extent, but who has to control her emotions in order to conduct the labour skilfully.

Whether or not the stillbirth is anticipated, you will probably be reassured by the baby's normal appearance if you do decide to hold him. Holding the baby can help you come to terms with his death and to understand his reality as a person. When you remember and grieve for him, he will not be an unseen 'fantasy baby'. You may prefer to be left alone together with the baby for a short time.

You may wish to recognize the baby's individuality by giving him a name. Unpleasant though it is, you will have to register the birth and the death of your child. There is often a registrar of births and deaths at the maternity hospital and the nursing staff will help you with the arrangement. You will need to discuss funeral arrangements and the hospital staff will again be able to help you contact a local funeral director.

Attitudes to stillbirth

Some people think that after a stillbirth the parents should forget all about it and think about other things. This rarely succeeds in erasing painful memories and can interrupt the process of grieving. Mourning is the natural, normal response to loss and there are no short cuts to by-pass the experience.

In hospital you may prefer to be in a single room, away from other mothers and their newborn babies. If there is no single room available, you may be put in a ward containing a number of other mothers who are separated from their babies for one reason or another, so that you do not have to bear this deprivation alone.

Some bereaved mothers feel that the hospital staff are not interested in them. This is very far from the truth. Often the staff desperately want to help but do not know what to do. They may feel that they are intruding or interfering in a private grief if they spend too much time with you; they may feel they have failed you by delivering a stillborn baby, even if the stillbirth was inevitable. Share your grief with them and, if you wish, particularly with the midwife who attended you in labour. She, too, will be mourning and will be under the strain of presenting a normal face to the other patients.

Try to use the stressful days after a stillbirth to express your grief and to begin the slow process of healing. Be considerate, in your distress, of those friends and relations who sympathize deeply but do not know how to respond or to help you. If, in later conversation, people laboriously steer clear of the subject of your baby's death, their usual motive will be that of not wishing to bring back your painful memories and of not appearing to be inquisitive. They are not avoiding the subject because they do not care.

You may find it helpful to talk to someone who has ex-perienced a stillbirth, and who can offer first-hand understand-ing and guidance.

Some hints about twins

A few general ideas

The mother who has learned how to relax completely and how to use only those muscles necessary for each task is at a tremen-dous advantage in coping with twins. If you can get one hundred per cent value out of each minute of rest and avoid becoming flustered and panicky as jobs pile up, you will have fresh energy to cope even though you are bound to get very tired at times. Correct posture and working habits learned during pregnancy will enable you to avoid backache and the general weariness that comes from poor posture. It is most important that you remember to do your postnatal exercises.

Plan ahead to get a lying-down rest each day, and get a couple of really early nights each week even though it means waking to feed the babies. Try to adopt a relaxed attitude to the problems you encounter. All new babies really need is plenty of milk whenever they want it, cleanish clothes, an occasional wash, and lots of loving. With twins it is easy to aim at standards which are too high for everyone's comfort.

It is wise, not extravagant, to spend money on help in the house, and on disposable nappies or a nappy service, or a fully automatic washing machine. A tumble drier is perhaps the most useful of all. There is no need to buy any elaborate baby equipment. Second-hand twin prams are cheap, but you will need another cheap pram or carrycot on wheels after the first six weeks or so, since the babies will keep each other awake. A folding twin pram/push-chair with separate back-rests is very handy for shopping and outings. If you have to take the twins on a weekly shopping expedition, it may be helpful to choose a shopping area which is pedestrianized or has wide pavements, or to go to a large 'superstore' (preferably with a crêche where the babies can be supervised) where everything is under one roof.

At first you will want to be able to get to know each baby separately, so it is much better not to have them both awake and crying at the same time if it can be avoided, and then you are less likely to become harrassed. Handle the babies as much as possible; you can never cuddle two babies as much as you could cuddle one. If you wish, take the babies to bed with you for an afternoon rest, making little nests for them in your bed, well free of blankets and pillows.

If you watch and closely observe your babies you will find that even identical twins are very different. It is this personal individuality which it is important to respect, loving each child for himself alone, not even for what he is in the family (the youngest or the eldest or one of the twins) or for what he might be if he were good all the time, but for himself, just as he is.

If possible have more clothing than you think you will need for the twins, even if they are cast-offs, so that when things really pile up you do not have to bother about washing and drying. It helps if the babies' – and the family's – clothes are made of drip-dry fabrics.

As they grow older many twins develop means of communication with each other which by-pass words, or even a special language which only the two of them understand. One child can be very distressed if a parent smacks the other, and on the whole this is best avoided.

Try not to leave the twins alone too often to amuse one another. Like all babies and children, they need the stimulus of frequent contact with an adult to help them develop skills in speech and social development.

You are bound to need means of keeping the babies within

a confined range. There are several forms of baby bouncer on the market and one or two of these hung out of harm's way in the kitchen will be useful for short periods after about four to six months. A playpen is almost essential. Once they are mobile, a light webbing harness on each baby can be quickly clipped in place on the high chair. In the garden you may wish to fence off a safe area using plastic-coated railing or plastic-coated strong wire netting.

You probably run more risk of accidents with two babies than with one, simply because you are busy and rushed. So plan ahead so that they cannot possibly topple out of highchairs or roll off beds.

Breastfeeding twins

Start breastfeeding as soon after birth as possible. Feed at least three-hourly at first, beginning with short feeds of about three minutes for each baby, and building up to about ten minutes each. Frequent feeding of both babies stimulates the breasts enough to supply milk for both babies. If you feed only one baby the stimulation is less and the breasts supply only enough milk for one baby.

Don't worry about timings: remember each baby is an individual and one may take longer to feed than the other. Many mothers have found it better to keep one breast for one baby rather than swop round at each feed. Each baby builds up his own supply on his own breast so that individual fluctuations of appetite can be catered for. You may feel a little 'lop-sided' at times if they vary much in demand, but it seems to settle down evenly after a couple of weeks.

You may find it easier to feed the babies separately at first so that you get to know each one as an individual and learn how to handle them and how to relax and enjoy feeding them. You may want to continue feeding your twins separately or you may find it easier to feed them together once you get the hang of it.

There are real advantages in feeding simultaneously. It takes less time when older children are around, less time at night, and

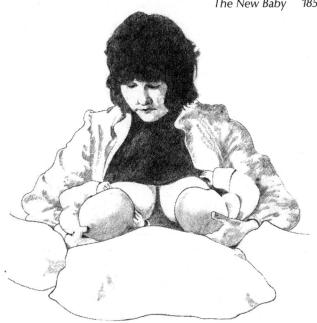

Breastfeeding twins simultaneously

is an advantage if both babies wake up hungry at the same time. A settee is the most comfortable place to feed your babies like this. You will need three pillows or cushions and something to wipe up dribbles. Place one pillow, to support their backs, on either side of where you intend to sit. Lay one baby safely on the settee and, holding the other baby in your arms, sit down, placing the third pillow on your lap. Lay one baby on each side, on his back, with the two heads close together on the pillow on your lap, so that their heads are just below your breasts. You may then hold the babies to the breast with your cupped hands under their heads, or adjust the pillow on your lap to support their heads. This leaves your hands free to wind each baby by turning him on to his tummy on the pillow where he may wind himself, or by raising him gently to your shoulder while the other continues feeding.

There may be times when you need to build up your milk supply, so feed every two or three hours for a day or so. Remember to eat and drink plenty yourself. (Your calorie output will be increased by at least 1,500 calories in the form of milk production.)

Bottle-feeding twins

Make sure that both babies get sufficient cuddling and enough of your handling and attention. Don't be tempted to hand one twin for feeding to anyone who happens to be around. As far as possible make feeding your job and use all the help you can for other chores. Simultaneous feeding means simultaneous hunger. It is much easier to get the babies going roughly one behind the other so there is time to get to know each one separately, and to have a hand free for a toddler.

If the twins are very tiny and need 2–3 hourly feeds you may find that you have to feed them together or you will literally never stop feeding. If you are feeding alone at night you will probably find that you will never get any sleep if you demand-feed entirely. Wake the second baby after finishing the first. If your husband is willing to get up at night to help with feeding you might find doing alternate nights each is better than both being up at every feed, or you could do alternate feeds each.

It is possible to bottle-feed two babies together by yourself. Sit on a bed or settee and prop one baby in the corner supported by cushions, holding his bottle in your left hand; cuddle the second baby with his head in the crook of your right arm, your right arm reaching in front of him to hold his bottle. This ensures that one baby gets some cuddling and you can alternate the one you hold at each feed.

Try not to get into the habit of propping both babies on cushions and just holding the bottles. This means that the babies miss out on close contact with you, and the temptation to prop up the bottles as well and get on with seemingly urgent tasks is great. This is a really dangerous thing to do because the babies can easily choke.

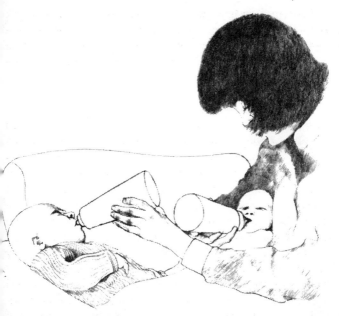

Bottle-feeding twins simultaneously

Make up feeds for 24 hours at a time and refrigerate them; it saves time and there is much less chance of contamination. A plastic bucket or bread bin makes a good sterilizing unit for the number of bottles you will be using.

Solid foods

When you introduce solid foods it is easiest to place the babies' high chairs close together (but not so close that they smother each other with food) and feed them alternately out of one bowl, either with the same spoon or with a spoon in each hand. Twins soon learn to feed each other, and each may find it simpler to put food in the other's mouth rather than his own!

Some mothers of twins, in an understandable attempt to save time, make the mistake of feeding their children exclusively on manufactured baby foods long after they could cope with

ordinary meals. You will save money, and help the twins' adjustment to eating solid foods, if you give them small portions of
the family's meals, puréed, mashed, or chopped as appropriate.

Adopted babies

Adoption is a large subject which can only be touched on
briefly, so mention is made here of only a few points which
adoptive parents have found to be of particular importance or
to be less well covered in the existing literature. There are a number of books available from public libraries outlining legal
procedures and discussing in full various practical and emotional
factors which couples considering adoption would do well to
think over before they approach an adoption agency. Once in
contact with an agency (or with your local authority) you will, of
course, have the help and support of the social worker handling
your case and of the health visitor when a baby finally arrives.

The first few days

It is difficult to generalize about adopted babies because they
are individuals who respond to life in their own very personal
ways. Frequently, however, they do have a rather different start
to life from the majority, arriving at the home of their adoptive
parents after a period in hospital and often after some weeks or
even months with foster parents. A baby is very sensitive to his
environment from birth onwards and may well show some
distress for a few days after his arrival at his adoptive parents'
home. He will have come to depend for comfort and reassurance on his foster mother and will be accustomed to the sights
and sounds of daily life in her home, so do not be surprised if
the baby who – you had been assured – was a model of good
behaviour, is at first restless and distressed. Natural parents
often have a similar experience on returning home with their
new babies! This will be an anxious time for you if this is your first
baby so, like other mothers, you will need to give as much time
as you can spare to relaxing and enjoying the baby and put your

own need to rest before the demands of housekeeping. If after a few days your baby still seems unduly troubled, your health visitor will be glad to give you guidance and reassurance, and you may well find that sharing your own maternal experience with friends and relatives or with the members of the NCT postnatal support group is a great aid in bolstering your morale.

From your point of view the arrival of your long-awaited baby may come as a bit of a shock. You may be taking this small stranger into your family after the briefest of introductions and without nine months' biological preparation which to the natural mother often seems over-long. Even if you are sure, within yourself, that you have great wells of maternal love just waiting to be released, your emotions in the hours following the baby's arrival may savour more of panic and a feeling that the world has turned a somersault, than of glowing motherly pride. Some adoptive parents feel that a little previous contact with their baby – a couple of visits to the foster home, for instance – helped them to ease themselves more gently into their new role, and gave the wife the chance to begin to see herself as the baby's mother. A husband too, may be unsure that he will be able to love someone else's child as well as his own, so he might also appreciate the opportunity to get to know the baby step by step. It might, therefore, be sensible to ask your social worker if one or two preliminary visits to the foster parents could be arranged.

You will soon come to know your baby intimately and as you do your love for each other will grow; indeed many natural mothers only 'fall in love' with their babies gradually over the early weeks, so do not feel ashamed if it turns out to be a gradual process for you.

Breastfeeding an adopted baby

Sometimes an adoptive mother longs to experience the close, loving relationship which can come from nursing a baby at the breast. It may come as a surprise to her to hear that this is not physiologically impossible, even for a woman who has never been pregnant. The stimulation of the breast by suckling can be sufficient to trigger off the secretion in the mother's body of the hormone prolactin, responsible for the production of breast milk. Trying to breastfeed an adopted baby is very hard work, but it can be very rewarding. A woman who has not recently given birth will probably not be able to fulfil all her baby's nutritional needs because her breasts have not been stimulated by pregnancy; nonetheless it is often possible to build up a milk supply after persuading the baby to suckle at an initially dry breast. And there lies the catch: although some babies will suck anything with gusto, most find it unrewarding to suckle at an unproductive breast (for a period varying from a few days to several weeks) before even a trickle of milk appears. A Lact-Aid, a gadget marketed in the USA which was designed by an adoptive father to help his wife to overcome this difficulty, is available from the NCT or La Leche League International. It consists, very simply, of a bag for the milk formula which is suspended round the mother's neck on a cord, to which is attached a length of very fine tube which lies against the breast to end at the mother's nipple. The baby can then receive his milk supply while suckling at the breast, giving him a reward for his efforts which will make him work harder. It is not so simple and straightforward to use as a baby's bottle, and is an awkward shape for cleaning, so it might not be worth the extra trouble for a baby who will suckle at breast or bottle without preference. Unlike a normal lactation, breastfeeding an adopted baby will involve a mother in more rather than less work: a factor which might deter someone who has other children in the family or who feels that it is going to take her all her time to care for her baby anyway. If, however, you feel that the mutual pleasure of nursing and the benefit to the baby that even a small amount of breast milk would bring would repay your initial effort, you are advised to contact the NCT some time before a baby is offered to you, to seek further advice, and to arrange for a counsellor to be in touch to give you help and support after the baby's arrival. You may also like to discuss the matter with your social worker, who might be able to arrange for you to have a very young baby, since one who has become accustomed to a bottle over a number of weeks will be much less likely to take to the breast than a relatively new baby.

The older baby

If you are adopting an older baby, or a toddler, breastfeeding will not be a consideration, but developing a loving bond between you will be equally important. The newcomer may be wary of you at first and may seem to reject you at precisely those times when you most want to give him your comfort and love. If you are patient and respect his feelings, he will soon come to trust you; though having gained you, he will be particularly anxious not to let you slip. He may panic in your absence and be, for a while, unusually timid about venturing far from your side. It is tempting for parents to feel that these and other difficulties are peculiar to their child because he is adopted, but many natural parents have in special circumstances had similar experiences with their children. Once again, do not hesitate to discuss your problems with other people.

Existing children's reactions

The busiest adoptive mother will be the one whose baby joins an existing family of children. Your previous experience will, of course, stand you in good stead, but you must reckon that your other child or children – far from being extra helpful – may well be a little extra demanding of your time and patience for a while, in particular the one who was the 'baby' of the family before. If they are old enough, they will be aware to some extent of the adoption procedure and will be excited and proud to tell their friends about 'our adopted baby'. You must be careful not to give them to understand that the arrangement is permanent until the adoption is finalized, otherwise they will be greatly distressed if the baby has to be returned to his natural mother and it may make them wonder if their own place in the family is secure. It would be as well to decide, right from the start, how much you intend to let your children (or anyone else) know about your baby's previous history, bearing in mind that what you tell your children will soon be known to all the world! They will be satisfied with a few quite simple facts and there is no need to give them detailed information which would be better written down and put away for safe keeping until your adopted child is older. Don't delay in committing details of an adopted baby's background to paper; even months afterwards you will find it impossible to sort out in your mind between what your social worker actually told you and what you deduced from information you were given.

Consideration towards adoptive parents

Lastly, a word for those of you reading this section who are not and do not expect to be adoptive parents. Please be especially considerate of anyone you encounter who is in the process of adopting a baby. The procedure itself is long and arduous, and is by no means over when the baby comes home, as it may be many months before the adoption is finalized and the parents can at last relax and get rid of the feeling of being eternally 'on approval'. Sometimes they may have had to face criticism from their wider family (it is natural enough, for instance, for grandparents to be anxious for the welfare of their other grandchildren when a baby or especially a toddler is brought into an existing family), and they will be particularly appreciative if you give the newcomer a warm welcome and show yourself ready to share in their joy and pleasure. Finally, a childless couple will have experienced much sorrow and stress because of their infertility, which will not be dispelled immediately by the new arrival, however delightful he may be. His mother will still feel to some extent that she missed the experience of pregnancy and giving birth and will long to know about the baby's birth and what took place before his arrival in her home. While she needs and will welcome the company of other new mothers, she might not wish to be regaled with the saga of your 'birth experience'.

THE NEW PARENTS

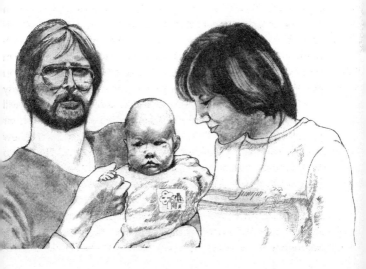

Introduction

The time immediately after the birth of a first baby is traditionally one for rejoicing, when grandparents and friends rally round and the new family becomes the centre of attention. Sometimes, however, the parents feel too stressed and unsure of themselves to enjoy these early days when everyone else seems so blissfully delighted. The relationship in the first six weeks or so between a mother and her new baby is very like the early days of a courtship or a honeymoon. Little drawbacks become magnified out of all proportion, while the pleasures are heightened into elation. It is a time of emotional extremes when your moods may swing from wonder and joy to helplessness and despair – all over things which, rationally, should cause you little concern. Be prepared for this, and enjoy the emotional 'highs' in all their intensity.

Here are a few practical points worth bearing in mind:

1. As a new mother, you need to eat sensibly to keep strong and active, and to maintain your milk supply if you are breastfeeding.

2. Just as pregnancy may call for adjustments in your sexual life, so the period of change after the baby is born can also affect your lovemaking – particularly if you have had an episiotomy and are apprehensive.

3. While most women adapt very well to motherhood, a small number, through no fault of their own, suffer from postnatal depression in varying degrees of severity. Medical help should always be sought for this condition. It can be treated and should never be a cause for shame or embarrassment.

4. Caring for a small baby can be an isolating experience, particularly if you live a long way from other members of your family or know few people in your neighbourhood. NCT groups throughout the country run informal systems for postnatal support, for women who seek this type of self-help and companionship.

5. It is important that the needs of each member of the new family are satisfied and respected. Mother, father, and children all have interdependent demands and you should work consciously to balance them, so that one person's desires do not become dominant.

Diet after the baby arrives

A good diet is important to keep a new mother healthy and thus able to look after her baby. Every new mother needs to eat well to have enough energy. If you are breastfeeding, you need to eat more to produce milk; even if you are bottle-feeding you need regular balanced meals or you will become over-tired and perhaps depressed. Eating something every two-and-a-half to three hours will help to raise the blood sugar level and keep depression at bay. For details of sources of essential nutrients, see p. 36.

Diet during breastfeeding

The breastfeeding mother is, indeed, eating for two. You will need more food than when you were pregnant. A baby consumes, on average, 600 calories a day.

Human milk is composed of protein, fat, carbohydrate (a special sugar called lactose), minerals, and vitamins. The protein can be provided by eating an extra 45 g (1½ oz) of meat or cheese or an extra half-pint of milk. The other nutrients in human milk can be made from carbohydrates: bread, potatoes, cereals, etc. Minerals and vitamins pass directly to the baby, so the mother's diet must contain enough for both of them.

If you are breastfeeding, your body will make milk for your baby before taking out your own nourishment, so protect your own health as well as your baby's by eating a well-balanced diet. Your milk supply is maintained by eating enough calories and by eating frequently. Do not miss meals, for you are making milk all the time. If your milk supply decreases, eat an extra snack or two; the supply may adjust itself within a few hours. If you feel tired or depressed, eat small amounts more often, to keep up your blood sugar level. If you feel ill and go off your food, with a resultant reduction of milk, don't worry: it will increase again as soon as you resume your normal diet.

Forbidden foods?

Is there any food a breastfeeding mother cannot eat? Generally speaking, no – you can eat what you fancy. The food is broken down by your digestive system and cannot get directly into the milk to affect the baby. (Drugs, on the other hand, pass directly into the milk, so consult your doctor about medicines.) Babies do not usually react adversely to any food that their mothers eat while producing breast milk. Eat whatever you were eating during pregnancy, and avoid an excessive intake of new foods – a sudden spicy meal or too much fruit or chocolate. If you do not normally eat a particular food, try a small amount of a moderately seasoned portion first. Seasonal fruits may need 'breaking in' in this way. Do not avoid fruit, however. Both you and the baby need the vitamin C, and it helps to prevent constipation. You need not avoid alcohol either; just drink in moderation.

Breastfeeding mothers get thirsty. You will need to drink more fluids than usual, and especially while feeding the baby. Any fluid will do; just follow your thirst and taste. Milk and stout are often recommended, but there is nothing magical about them. Milk does not make milk; it is simply a very good source of calories, protein, calcium, and other nutrients. Too much coffee or tea, incidentally, may reduce your milk supply, so drink these in moderation while establishing breastfeeding. Do not force yourself to drink, especially if you are worried that you haven't enough milk. There is some evidence to show that when mothers are forced to drink more water than they want, they produce less milk.

Losing weight

You will probably be 3–6 kg (7–14 lb) over your pre-pregnancy weight after the baby is born. This is nature's way of providing a reserve to make milk. Do not try to diet while establishing breastfeeding – you are more likely to reduce the milk supply and exhaust yourself. The extra few pounds generally disappear during the first few months of looking after a new baby – and breastfeeding helps this process – or else after weaning the baby. Be sure to do postnatal exercises so that your muscles will be back into shape in preparation for your weight loss later. Sometimes pregnancy alters the body's metabolism and you may need to go on a slimming diet after weaning. Eating well, but not to excess, should be your rule while your baby is still new and you need all the energy you can get.

Sex after the baby is born

After the drama of labour it is wonderful to hold your newborn child in your arms and to realize that you are suddenly parents, even though it hardly seems believable. The sense of having as a couple shared the making of the baby can be very strong, and many couples find that the feeling of sharing continues through-out parenthood. Others, however, find that the baby becomes the focus of so much attention that its parents have trouble relating to each other except as parents, or that they spend so much time paying attention to the baby that they make too little time for themselves. It is rather like having a house-guest: when even a weekend visitor comes, for instance, couples can quickly find that they seldom see each other alone or when not pre-occupied with the guest's needs or with the alterations the visit makes to their usual pattern of life. And, depending on the guest, you can find it easy or difficult to adjust. With congenial friends staying overnight after a special meal and relaxing evening, you may feel perfectly happy to leave dirty dishes for the morning and to retire to bed and make love just as you always do. Whereas with your parents-in-law you might not feel quite so uninhibited, either about leaving the dishes or about making love ('Not tonight, in case the bed creaks and disturbs them'). You become the model host and hostess, not your usual selves. In the same way, many couples react to the birth of their first baby by beginning to see themselves as the baby's mother and father more often than as a loving couple. But labour does not mysteriously turn a woman into a Mother Earth figure with no sexual desires, and fatherhood does not transform a husband into a man with only paternal feelings.

Many adjustments have to be made after the birth of a baby, and family relationships all shift in subtle ways as a new generation of parents – and grandparents – is created. The arrival of second and subsequent babies also causes changes.

The birth of a baby can place stress on even a happy marriage if the wife believes she is an undesirable drudge or the husband feels neglected in favour of the baby. They may both feel they can never recapture the romance of courtship and early marriage and the spontaneity of lovemaking.

Traditional attitudes

As with sex in pregnancy, traditions of many kinds linger on over the behaviour of new parents. In some cultures the woman receives special protection: she may be fed special foods and treated in a ritual manner. In other cultures, the father is thought to need special attention: in the custom known as the 'couvade', for instance, *he* goes to bed and is cosseted during or after his wife's labour. In this country, some women feel that they cannot take up their normal lives until after they have been 'churched'.

In many societies one of these traditions is a ban on intercourse for a specified period after childbirth. The reasons given vary, including fear of injuring the vagina or introducing infection to the uterus, and bear little relation to evidence of when any one woman feels physically capable of intercourse, which may be as soon as a week after a normal delivery. The length of advised abstinence differs from country to country: for instance, six weeks in the USA and three in France. In Britain opinions vary: some doctors say you should wait until after the six-week check, while others say you should be sure to recommence before the six-week check so that you can raise any problems at it.

Nevertheless, although a woman may be physically ready for sex very shortly after the birth of her child, she often feels in need of a period of sexual respite. However deeply she loves her husband, she may dislike the thought of making love or may lose interest once lovemaking has started. Almost without exception she will want her husband to give her extra care and attention. This may be a time when other expressions of love are appropriate.

Too tired

The old excuse 'I'm too tired' may be only too true for the new mother. Her day is filled with new experiences and new responsibilities so that in bed she longs only for the oblivion of sleep. She may be so tense and pre-occupied that she is unable to get into the mood of mutual giving and receiving necessary for happy lovemaking. (Clearing her mind by doing her breathing and relaxation techniques may be helpful.) The baby may be waking her regularly at night for feeds, and she may not have managed to sleep during the day, despite good intentions. Finally, her husband may not be as sympathetic and helpful as she would wish, forgetting that sex at night is for her closely linked with his behaviour during the day.

Sensitive spots

Making love after childbirth can be pretty uncomfortable. The natural vaginal lubrication may be absent at this time and the vagina itself may feel taut and dry. You may both find it helpful if the woman uses a lubricating jelly or cream (for instance a contraceptive cream or one sold for keeping the nipples supple) in her vagina and smoothes some on her partner's penis before penetration.

If the woman has had stitches she will not only be sore, she will (unless she is a paragon of self-control) have negative memories of the episiotomy and suturing process and may subconsciously recoil from having such a sensitive place touched again. In the days immediately following the episiotomy the stitches may only 'prickle', or they may be so painful that practically every bodily movement pulls them. After this has passed, there is often a tender lump along the line of the incision for the next few months. Any pressure against this will be unpleasant and may be emphasized if the woman tenses and draws back in apprehension when her husband tries to enter her.

When making love after there has been a tear or an episiotomy it is important not only to make sure that there is enough lubrication but also to choose a position in which the penis presses on the clitoris and front wall of the vagina rather than against the tender area at the back. The woman will find it helpful to guide the man inside her while she deliberately releases her pelvic floor muscles. If intercourse continues to be painful in spite of consideration and gentle lovemaking, she should consult her obstetrician.

After birth the woman may find clitoral stimulation particularly enjoyable and should help her husband to discover exactly what gives her the most pleasure. You may both find that positions which before giving birth were perfectly acceptable are now associated by the woman with obstetric procedures and are consequently quite off-putting to her. Experimentation may be necessary until the memories fade.

If the wife is breastfeeding, her husband should be careful not to put pressure on her sensitive breasts. She will be especially milky and uncomfortable at night if the baby unexpectedly sleeps longer than usual between feeds. Sometimes when the breasts become sexually aroused they leak milk. To minimize this it is best to make love soon after a feed. Once again, you may need to try different positions for sex.

One, or both, of you may be inhibited about making love if the baby is in the same room. Put the child behind a screen or move him to another room.

Contraception

You may worry about starting another baby very soon, since contraceptives are not usually prescribed until the postnatal examination at six weeks. Breastfeeding usually inhibits ovulation but not always, so it is very unwise to rely on it as a form of contraception. The wife may not want to take the Pill if she is breastfeeding, but if she does she should make sure it is the 'mini-Pill'. Her milk supply will probably be reduced for a couple of days after commencing it, but will pick up again if she feeds more frequently for 48 hours.

The man may use a sheath, but this may cause discomfort to a dry and tender vagina and will prevent the woman feeling her husband's ejaculation. If the wife used a cap before the baby was conceived she will find that it will now be too small, but smeared liberally with spermicide it should provide adequate protection until she can obtain another. If she has no cap, the best answer may be to insert a lot of spermicide into the vagina, near the cervix, with the applicator provided.

The pelvic floor

Regaining strength and tone in the pelvic floor muscles is important after childbirth, though it may take six to eight weeks to achieve. Slackness of the pelvic floor muscles can lead not only to prolapse and stress incontinence but to difficulties in lovemaking, when the wife cannot make the subtle gripping movements of the vagina which are so pleasurable. The pelvic floor may sag if the woman has a bad cough, strains because of constipation, or is depressed and miserable. She feels as if her insides are dropping out, may get low backache and feel very weary. Doing the simple pelvic floor exercises learned in pregnancy can help break into this pattern of feeling unwell. Pelvic floor rehabilitation exercises are described on pp. 123–4.

The tone of the woman's pelvic floor muscles can be assessed by her husband if she contracts them rhythmically when they make love. In this way she can strengthen and improve them not only for supporting the uterus and bladder, but for giving and receiving much pleasure in intercourse.

Further postnatal exercises

The new mother also needs to strengthen her abdominal wall and the muscles which support her breasts. For the latter, hold your wrists with either hand, elbows raised above shoulder level, and while maintaining the grip on the wrists, push your hands towards your elbows with a jerking movement. The abdominal muscles can be strengthened by lying on your back on the floor and lifting your head to look at your toes. As the muscles improve you will be able to lift yourself to a sitting position and then slowly down again. DO NOT lift both legs in the air – the movement must be head towards feet, not feet towards the head. Also DO NOT do the exercise with your feet hooked under a wardrobe, or other solid piece of furniture. To slim your waist, lie on your back with your knees bent up and feet flat on the bed and drop and raise your knees together from side to side, both to the right and up, then both to the left and up. These exercises may be repeated five times and done twice a day, then increased to ten times.

Postnatal support

In providing services to support the mother with a new baby, the National Childbirth Trust does not imply that everyone will need – or wish – to make use of them. If you are in good health, with a thriving and contented baby, and comfortably settled in your home, with friends and family near at hand, you may well feel that life has never been better! You may welcome the release from the routines of your former employment and, despite the ceaseless round of feeding and washing that babies entail, find great pleasure not only in your baby but in a variety of home-based activities for which you had little leisure when you were out at work. You may, or may not, wish to take advantage of the additional contact available through NCT postnatal support groups, where your calmness and general *joie de vivre* may be a great help to those who are lonely or experiencing problems.

Alas, not everyone finds life with a new baby so congenial. Not infrequently, the birth of her first baby heralds a time of great loneliness for a woman. Couples may move to a new home in another district when they start a family; while others have had limited opportunity to make friends in their neighbour-hood, when they were both out at work all day. Babies (lovable though they may be) cannot compensate for the variety of stimuli provided by, say, a day at the office, and chatting about the weather with the girl at the cash desk of the supermarket is a poor exchange for sharing daily life with friends and colleagues who really know and appreciate you. NCT postnatal support may be particularly helpful in this kind of situation.

Friendly support

The opportunity to meet other mothers with babies over a cup of coffee is offered by the NCT in many areas, to help the new mother overcome her loneliness and make new friends. These gatherings are usually held in members' homes, weekly, fort-nightly, or monthly, but may take the form of a baby club in a church hall or similar accommodation. If you have attended NCT antenatal classes you will be informed if such arrange-ments exist in your own locality, but such get-togethers (unless they are specifically 'class reunions') are open to any new mother, who, having contacted her local Branch or Group to find out time and place, can be assured of a warm welcome. Additional social activities are organised in many parts of the country and such mutual services as baby-sitting clubs have proved very popular.

Most Branches and Groups produce regular newsletters with articles of interest to parents of a baby or toddler, and valuable information about local services such as the facilities offered in shops and public places for feeding and changing babies, sports facilities for mothers with young families, and mother and toddler clubs. In fact, NCT members prove a mine of information on everything that concerns the new mother, from knitting patterns to the current local rate for baby-minders if you are to return to work.

Help in a crisis

The best laid plans for joyful parenthood can be upset by a sudden crisis on the domestic front. In any part of the country where there are NCT members, you can expect to find people who are responsive to your needs when an emergency arises, and in a number of larger Branches and Groups a postnatal support secretary can call upon volunteers who are organized to give help in a crisis. For instance, a 'milk run' may be set up for a mother who is expressing breast milk for her hospitalized baby, or a 'chauffeur' provided for someone who has to keep hospital appointments but is unfit to drive or travel on public transport. Not infrequently, a mother who is unwell may welcome temporary assistance with shopping and household chores, or with ferrying another child to nursery school or play-group. Postnatal support 'helpers' may come into antenatal classes to explain the services offered and may, in addition, call in when you and the baby are home from hospital, as a reminder that they are there to hand if needed. However, all such post-natal services are organized on a local basis so there is no uniform pattern, and often no great degree of formality in the arrangements, which are, after all, only an extended form of good-neighbourliness.

In the early months, the majority of mothers experience at least some moments of depression, anxiety or extreme fatigue; for some the condition may be severe and long-lasting. At such a time it is hard to be out-going and to participate in such events as coffee mornings for new mothers, when it may require a superhuman effort merely to face the daily round. If you feel like this, you may find yourself shunning the company even of old friends and neighbours, especially if you sense their criticism of your apparent lethargy and inability to cope domestically. You may find comfort, at such a time, in the friendship of an NCT member who has perhaps herself had personal experience of postnatal depression, or has the personal qualities necessary to accept you, just as you are, in your present unhappiness.

In some situations there is of course every reason for distress. A baby may be sick, sometimes dying, or born with a handicap, in which case practical as well as emotional assistance may be required. However hard it may be for you to talk about your anxiety and grief, you should be able to expect from NCT members compassion and a readiness to be available when needed, to listen and support.

If the NCT is not listed in the local telephone directory, apply to Headquarters and you will be put in touch with an appropriate person.

Postnatal depression

Your baby has been born, you are surrounded by flowers and messages of congratulation – everything should be marvellous. The first couple of days after the birth have been filled with euphoria, now suddenly all you want to do is weep. You are obsessed with small details of your labour, where you feel somehow you failed; every whimper from the baby heralds a disaster; every word from the nurses brings you to the verge of tears.

This describes to some extent how you may feel shortly after the birth of your baby. It is usually called 'the third-day blues' and a large proportion of women experience the feeling. For the majority, it is soon over. However, some women may find that they are engulfed by depression for a time some days after they leave hospital, while a tiny minority experience such severe depression that they need special care.

Depression

Depression can mean different things to different people. For some it is a transient mood, and for others, a lasting emotiona experience usually associated with an important event in life Other people may think of depression as a shameful illness and a breakdown from normality. Perhaps depression can be described best as a part of life, ranging from the mood swings known to most people, to deep despair and mental disorder.

Postnatal depression

When birth is this big event in your life, a number of changes take place: the baby is born, you become a mother, your husband is transformed from lover to father, and a new family begins. These changes can expose you to considerable stress and how you cope depends on a complex interaction o factors. The stress can lead to strong feelings, some recognized others apparently coming from nowhere. If these feelings become too strong, they get 'switched off' and depression is experienced.

Birth   It is estimated that two-thirds of all women experience a degree of depression after childbirth. There seems some evidence that the birth itself – the quality of your antenata preparation, the attitudes of your medical attendants, the kind of delivery you have, whether or not the baby is left with you and how feeding is established – affects how you adapt to these changes, and how you see yourself in the new identity of mother. Yet depression may still occur with the best preparation and birth experience.

Hormonal causes   During pregnancy, the hormones in your body undergo significant changes in order to enable the baby to grow, to set labour in motion and to stimulate lactation. For example, progesterone (which, among its functions, is responsible for a feeling of well-being) increases production a hundredfold during pregnancy. This hormone ensures that the baby obtains adequate nourishment through the placenta which itself becomes an extra production centre. After the birth the placenta is discarded and a rapid drop in the production of progesterone takes place. The hormonal system then lives in a temporary state of imbalance. Many women experience 'third-day blues' or 'baby blues' in this period, with tears alternating with excitement and awe. These rapid and often bewildering changes of mood may last for a few days, but with loving care, understanding, and quiet confidence from your partner and attendants, you may find yourself settling down. The normal production of progesterone begins again as in the non-pregnant state. There are other hormonal influences and further implications of hormonal imbalance are currently being investigated.

Social and physical causes   For other women, the transition takes longer. The new mother leaves hospital with high expectations of herself. Sometimes she has not been married for long, often she may be living far from close friends and family. She may have had a good job in which she felt capable and financially independent. Motherhood seems a difficult role. Her skills no longer work. The baby cries, her partner comes home hungry and tired, she knows nobody to talk with during the day and the organization of time becomes chaotic. She becomes anxious and the baby responds with further crying and unsettled sleep. Physical fatigue sets in – somehow there is never enough time and sleep becomes an all-consuming need. She finds herself longing for old freedoms and for the bliss of the early days of the relationship. She tries again and again to sort it all out, but the secret eludes her. Everyone else seems to be coping: why isn't she? She looks tired and lethargic, and feels a sense of despair and loneliness, of being overwhelmed and losing herself. Sexually, she feels too tired to make love, and then realizes that she does not want to anyway, and takes this as proof of her inadequacy as a woman. She may try to explain to other people, but she may also give up, and retreat into apathetic silences or irritable flare-ups, feeling guilty and unlovable inside. Many men feel upset and bewildered if their wives behave in this way, though some may be able to perceive that the woman has been unable to adjust emotionally and physically to the new role of mother.

If you feel like this, you will probably be in a downward spiral of fatigue and loss of confidence. If your husband can see this and understand, he may be able to shift his own position by helping more, expecting less and showing you that he loves you and has faith in you. He should look for solutions which fit your temperament and needs, perhaps by arranging visits to or from someone, by feeding the baby at night for a week (even with a breastfed baby he can give an occasional bottle), by asking the doctor for sleeping tablets to help you, and by taking extra time off work so that he can help in a practical way and share your knowledge of how demanding a baby can be (most people don't realize how emotionally exhausting it may be to have a crying baby whom you can find no way of soothing). Extra sleeping time and outings together, and on your own without the baby, can help you to feel your way gradually into a more stable position. The anxiety lessens, the baby settles and the transition comes to an end. You can be yourself, *and* a mother, and your expectations are more realistic.

Non-understanding   Resolution of the problem is unfortunately not always so straightforward. Your husband may be genuinely bewildered and respond by telling you to 'pull yourself together', resulting in further tears and distress for you. It seems as if the birth has triggered off memories of old losses and as if you yourself crave the soothing care and attention of a mother. Responsibility becomes a burden and you may find it difficult to share the strength of your feelings, which may be quite horrifying to you. You may even find yourself wishing to harm the baby, which naturally fills you with shame and guilt. Your husband feels powerless. It is difficult for you both to imagine that any other couple could feel so despairing, and you are unable to share the pain with others or with one another. Communications break down.

Treatment

Family and community help   Depression which comes with a 'life event' progresses in a way which tends to be self-healing, and the experience can be a crucial point of growth towards maturity and a clearer picture of yourself and your family. This does not mean that the time of depression is any less painful, nor does it mean that it is a helpful response to say only that it will soon be all over. Active support during a time of depression is still essential. There are resources to help a family through the experience. If you have learned about depression in preparation classes, you can be aware of what is happening. The feelings can be shared and a survival campaign worked out. Preparation classes themselves give a network of supporting friends, and opportunities for postnatal occasions and individual counselling. In many areas The National Childbirth Trust runs classes which continue after the birth, when you return to your former class with your baby, and share your experiences. You are introduced to other mothers in your area, providing friendship and babysitting help. Such self-help groups can be invaluable to young parents (see 'Postnatal support', p. 204). The community itself helps where the wider family is no longer near enough to give practical and physical support.

Professional services   There are professional workers who can be consulted about postnatal depression. The health visitor who comes to see you at home can be sensitively understanding and supportive, with extra visits and practical encouragement. The general practitioner can assess the situation in your whole family. He can prescribe tranquillizers to help you to sleep and may suggest a course of anti-depressant pills, although, since an inability to cope is probably one reason for your depression, you may not be helped much by living in a drugged 'tranquillized' state all day which makes it difficult to look after yourself and the baby. Sometimes it is hard to find the right kind of help.

The health visitor and GP may seem to have little time to listen and explain, and you may trail off apologetically at the end of a wasted visit. In this kind of situation, it can help if your husband is present at the consultation. If you can both recognize what is happening and accept that you need help, you can usually find someone to share the problem. This does require a certain amount of courage but sometimes the right person appears in an unexpected guise. The deepest need does seem to be for warm accepting human contact at this time. There is a Social Services Department in every town where help may be available from a social worker. The Samaritan Service and MIND groups are other sources of help, and can be found in the telephone directory.

Mental disorder

There are some mothers who go further along the continuum of distress into mental disorder, when they act in unusual ways and become out of touch with reality. In this situation it is important that a doctor is called even without the woman's permission. She may need special care in a hospital, where she can be looked after with her baby until she can take over responsibility for herself again. Depression of this kind may have shown symptoms in earlier life. If this is known, a woman can have skilled therapy before the birth to minimize the subsequent situation and to establish a support system ready to go into action. Progesterone therapy has been shown to be helpful for some women.

Prevention

In our present state of knowledge, it would be foolish to think that all depression could be prevented. If depression is part of change and growth, perhaps the task is to accept it with information and understanding. By taking away some of the panic and fear of the unknown, inner resources can be mobilized more easily and sharing can take place. Preparation groups which cover the periods before and after the birth provide information, support and friendly faces as well as practical help. Knowledge of the local services and how to use them is important for all families. For a couple, it is important to establish trustworthy friendships before the birth of the baby if they cannot turn to the wider family, and to know how to contact a counsellor in the community.

The new family

Each new family must work out its own structure and relationships: words of advice in a book will make little difference to serious problems and will be unnecessary if everything instinctively goes well. However, in the time of change after the birth of a first baby, it can be easy to adopt patterns of behaviour which may cause stress later on, and to slip into habits which are hard to break even when commonsense tells you they are. Perhaps what follows may help you to nip such tendencies in the bud.

Family structure

When the new baby arrives he naturally becomes the focus of attention. This is good and inevitable but you should be careful to make sure that the baby does not become *too* important. All the members of your new family are equally valuable: the baby and his needs should fit into the existing family framework wherever possible. Don't change your lifestyle completely just because you are now parents – you are more than likely to come to resent the baby's intrusion into your settled ways. Fit in with his overwhelming needs – feed him when he is hungry, cuddle him when he is lonely, change his nappies when he is smelly. But, having satisfied these basic physical needs, start to satisfy your own while making allowances for his presence. If you want to make a journey, take him with you; if you need a break, leave him with a reliable baby-sitter; if you are invited to a party, take him too if practical. Accustom the child to a life full of new experiences, always buffered by your love and calmness, and you will lay good foundations for later. It is not kind, in the long run, to 'hibernate' for the sake of your young baby. You all miss a lot of fun and sharing.

It is possible to let the pendulum swing too far in the other direction and, instead of the baby being the boss, the parents are not realistic in making allowance for its dependence and needs. Knowing what small babies can and cannot do, and how they develop over the first months, is important. Just as it is not wise to change your entire lifestyle when a baby arrives, it is equally unwise to expect a baby to make no difference at all.

Couples will want to ensure that their own relationship does not get out of balance either. They are still husband and wife and not re-cast as 'the baby's father and mother'. Each will need to be careful not to presume on the other, and an honest sharing of feelings and tasks will make a great difference. At one end of the scale you may have a woman with a gentle doting husband who is so self-indulgent about her vulnerability as a mother that she tricks her partner into doing everything for her: what starts as constant requests for help can turn, over the months, into a full-blown matriarchy and exploitation of the husband's good nature. Heavy-handed patriarchs, at the other end of the scale, are not common nowadays, but if your husband shows this tendency in a way which you feel is damaging to the marriage or to the baby, use your skill and patience to divert him from this role. Couples whose relationship falls somewhere in the middle of these two extremes can still hurt one another thoughtlessly. It is easy to see how difficulties can arise from different viewpoints: the new mother may regard herself as 'being stuck at home all day looking after a demanding baby' and feel she deserves some looking after by her husband when he comes home – whereas the husband may feel he is quite justified in expecting meals ready without fail because his wife has 'nothing to do all day except look after a little baby'.

Sometimes a couple's longed-for baby becomes so precious

to them that in their eyes he changes from an ordinary little human being into a love object. He ceases to be a person, with mortal qualities and faults, and is a little idol whom they worship for their own gratification. Every need or imagined whim is indulged by the adoring parents, and the child becomes a greedy monster destined either for a later rude awakening or for lifelong unpopularity with his fellows. Because he is not treated like an ordinary person, the child misses the rough and tumble of normal growing-up and his grip on the world is unsound. The parents of such a child never really get to know him, either because they project all their fantasies on to him, or because they are so interested in their own feelings that they do not bother about his. For all concerned, the creation of a love object is unhealthy.

In an ideal world everyone would know their spouse so well that they would be able to predict how parenthood would affect them; but we don't always anticipate our own reactions, far less those of our partners. Husbands should not expect their wives to be transformed overnight into Mother Earth figures who can instinctively feed, pacify, and cherish a squalling new-born child. By the same token, wives should not expect their husbands to be bowled over by the minutiae of babyhood – nappies, feeds, and achievements – to the exclusion of everything else. There is more to life than nappy pails, but the woman who is too harrassed to realize this is in danger of neglecting her marriage. Equally the husband who disregards these matters, denying the importance of being a mother, also puts the marriage under stress.

Changing perspectives

Most parents, expectant or fulfilled, find that their ideas of entertainment and leisure-time pursuits change as they get used to thinking of themselves as a family with children instead of just a couple, so that far from grumbling about not being able to be as they were before, they are delighted to move into a new era in their lives and to share its pleasures and compensations.

Pregnancy and labour are great adventures, and parenthood progresses slowly enough to allow for gradual adaptation and immense pleasure not only in guiding the development and interests of your child but also in seeing the world afresh through his eyes.

Sharing

Share the babycare tasks which can be divided between you, but do this because you want equal loving contact with the baby and not because they are chores. Be realistic about sharing. In coping with night feeds, for instance, your husband may happily help by picking up the baby, but he need not be forced to share your broken nights if it makes difficulties: he cannot catnap at work, during the day, to make up the sleep deficit. He can make his contribution at another time, by helping with the housework, cuddling or bathing the baby, or changing nappies. Work out what suits you both best and enjoy your baby together.

Some people still think that babycare is 'woman's work' and this can cause problems. It may be that the new mother gets pleasure from feeling indispensible, or that she has old-fashioned ideas about gender roles. By monopolizing the baby she can frustrate her husband's desire to be a tender and caring father, and can hurt him very much. On the other hand, a new father may leave the children entirely to the mother, thus cutting himself off from them and from her. Parenthood is basically begun as a shared thing and should continue that way.

First-time parents should recognize that a significant proportion of their practical childcare techniques derives from how they themselves were brought up. It can be unsettling for two people who are perfectly happily married to discover how different these background experiences can be. You are well advised to talk with each other about this so that you don't unconsciously cause unnecessary strains by working on different assumptions. It is astonishing to discover the heated arguments which can arise over how to fold and fasten a nappy.

The tiniest matters will come under scrutiny, and probably won't show until mother, father, and baby are all at home at the same time. Then you realize the incredible variety of theories on child care and that the way your family did things was only one of many approaches.

If you as a couple have faced some of these choices, laughed at their seeming importance and begun to set your own ways of caring for your own baby, you will be off to a good start and will not be upset by people advising yet another approach.

Confidence

Have confidence in the way you handle your baby. He is part of you both, and you soon know him better than anyone else does. Once you have decided on a rough 'philosophy' for bringing up your child, support one another in it. Be true to your own convictions and don't feel bound by fashion or by family traditions.

Be patient with those who want to help you. The company of new parents, however confident and accomplished they are, brings out both the protective and the bossy instincts in other couples. You will never be at a loss for advice. Be tolerant and remember that you, in turn, will be tempted to treat other new parents in exactly the same way!

Your parents and older relatives will feel especially responsible for you and it may require almost superhuman efforts on their behalf not to bombard you with their worries and reminiscences. They may have unrealistically rosy ideas about how well they coped with you as a new baby. Respect their experience as parents (after all, you have thrived!) while treating their advice in the light of your own beliefs. Do not allow anyone to destroy your confidence in what you think is best, but be prepared to learn from all available sources. Remember, as far as childcare fashions go, there is nothing new under the sun.

Improvising

Don't try to keep up with the Joneses if you can't afford to. Set a fashion for self-help and eccentricity by buying second-hand equipment (wash it thoroughly before use), the minimum number of baby clothes (you may receive a lot as presents), and by spending your money on items like high quality terry nappies (or disposable ones, if you prefer), which will save time and effort later. If, as a housewife, you totter from one muddle to the next, it may be better to spend the Child Benefit Allowance on once-a-week domestic help rather than on a succession of baby-suits or as a supplement to the housekeeping funds.

Whole industries are created when manufacturers invent a 'need' for the babycare market. Take heart that the human race has survived until now with these 'needs' unsatisfied. Use your ingenuity for making labour-saving items. The possibilities for improvisation are endless: though safety must always be the prime factor in any do-it-yourself designs.

Resist impulse buys for the child and don't spend a lot of money on toys. Your baby is blissfully unaware of his material status – all he cares about is your loving, consistent care.

And finally . . .

If you have a bad birth experience, or can't (or don't want to) breastfeed, try not to feel guilty about it. You have not been responsible for what has happened, so guilt is quite out of place. To feel guilty about having needed medical technology and expertise during your labour is to deny the life-saving progress in obstetrics and paediatrics which has taken place in the last generation. And to feel guilty if you are repelled by the thought of breastfeeding your baby is wrong, too; it is a common feeling experienced by many other women.

Events rarely go according to the mental plan you conjure up beforehand. Your experiences in pregnancy, labour, and childcare, will inevitably turn out to be different from your anticipations. What matters is how you deal with the real experiences. Don't waste time and emotional energy feeling guilty or disappointed about the failure of your fantasies to stand up to reality.

Introducing The National Childbirth Trust (NCT)

Our organization was founded in 1956 to improve women's knowledge about childbirth and to promote the teaching of relaxation and breathing for labour. In the years of experience since then, we have learned from mothers of other needs surrounding the experience of pregnancy and parenthood, and we have widened our interests and our training courses in response.

The NCT is a growing and flexible organization, maintaining its primary interest in the importance of excellent antenatal preparation. Members come from all walks of life – professional, skilled, unskilled – and each offers particular knowledge which is relevant to the field of early parenthood. NCT work overlaps into many specialities: teaching, obstetrics, paediatrics, social work, and psychology, to name but a few. The NCT has advisers from many fields and is continually learning from them: a number of the advisers have contributed to sections in this book. We have found that the value of a multi-disciplinary organization cannot be overestimated in the field of parenthood.

Aims

The National Childbirth Trust aims to set and maintain high standards of antenatal education; to assess the needs of expectant mothers and new parents and to help to get these needs met; to press for informed choice for expectant parents; and to emphasize the need for good emotional support for women in labour.

Antenatal classes

When the NCT was founded, few books about childbirth were available, little encouragement was offered to mothers by the medical profession, and women who asked questions about physical changes during pregnancy and birth were often regarded as unnecessarily inquisitive or over-anxious. The NCT can claim to have had considerable influence in changing this attitude, so that now the woman who wishes to take the trouble to prepare herself to co-operate effectively both with her attendants and with her own body when she is giving birth, will usually receive help and encouragement. Whatever help is given should reinforce the idea of personal responsibility. A woman can take active steps to maintain her own health and that of her baby, and to prepare for her role as a mother.

In labour, a knowledge of relaxation and controlled breathing can be invaluable to all women, whatever the policy of each individual hospital with regard to drugs and obstetric aids. If the skills of relaxation and controlled breathing are taught in conjunction with a wide range of information about childbirth by teachers who want women to have an agreeable experience of giving birth, the benefits to parents and families can be profound. Preparation for husbands to work with their wives during pregnancy and labour and to gain an awareness of parenthood is also increasingly a part of NCT antenatal education.

Antenatal teachers and antenatal classes

Education offered to expectant parents should be relevant to their needs. The skill with which this is done will depend largely on the personality, ability, and training of the teacher. So one of our most important aims has been to devise a careful, comprehensive, and stimulating course of teacher training, based on a tutorial system, and to present it in such a way that it can be taken by women who are primarily occupied in bringing up their own children. They know what it feels like to be pregnant and to give birth, but they have learnt to listen as well as to teach. Classes are always informal, with opportunities for discussion as an integral part. Teachers, after their initial training, are provided with a study programme, frequent contact with other teachers who have between them a wide variety of professional and other background knowledge, and they are kept in touch with new ideas in education and in obstetric theory and practice.

Breastfeeding counselling

The decline in the skill and acceptance of breastfeeding had reached alarming proportions by 1970, when only one in ten mothers in Britain breastfed her baby. The NCT at that stage decided to offer training to women who had experience of breastfeeding and who wished to help other women to succeed in feeding their babies naturally. The value of these 'breast-feeding friends' was quickly proved, since in many cases they fulfilled a role which used to be undertaken by mothers and grandmothers in a more static society. The NCT now offers study facilities for those mothers who wish to act as breast-feeding counsellors, offering non-medical advice and support to nursing mothers. The Breastfeeding Promotion Group is an active group within the NCT.

Postnatal support

Comprehensive education for parenthood has always been the NCT's primary aim, and offering support in the postnatal period is recognized as a corollary to this first goal. We hope by doing this to help to reduce the incidence of depression, anxiety, and loneliness in young mothers, and to reduce the development of dangerous tensions in the family.

Education in schools

The NCT's experience with thousands of young parents has made us concerned over the lack of information about human reproduction given in our educational system. Those NCT members who are experienced schoolteachers have realized the significance of birth as a part of sex education and have seen the need for discussing breastfeeding as a part of childcare.

Some of our antenatal teachers have been invited to schools to give talks on birth. The NCT now offers study days on ways of teaching about birth and breastfeeding in school programmes, for teachers and parents.

Study events, conferences, and study groups

The NCT holds frequent study days and weekend seminars on many aspects of education for childbirth, parenthood, and breastfeeding. From time to time internationally-known experts are featured at special lectures and study days. Regional conferences, small conferences for specialist groups, and NCT branch conferences are also held. Interdisciplinary groups are convened to study particular aspects of childbirth, and may publish papers on the basis of their discussions.

Publications and other services

The NCT has produced a series of leaflets for expectant parents, which are revised to keep up to date with obstetric and antenatal developments. The NCT sells a range of books, records and tapes on pregnancy, preparation for birth, and breast-feeding.

The NCT markets the unique Mava maternity and nursing brassiere, carefully designed in 40 sizes to meet the needs of pregnant and nursing mothers. Other products, for babies and parents, are also available.

A hire service for electric breast pumps is organized to help mothers of sick or premature babies to provide breast milk.

Local branches of the NCT in most parts of the United Kingdom offer antenatal classes, breastfeeding counselling, and postnatal support.

For details of local representatives, publications, and other services, please apply to NCT Headquarters, 9 Queensborough Terrace, London W2 3TB, telephone 01-229-9319/9310.

Further reading

(In each case the date given is that of first publication)

ANTENATAL

Brant, Herbert & Margaret: *Dictionary of Pregnancy, Childbirth and Contraception* (Corgi, 1975)

Burns, Lois: *Your Baby and Your Figure* (Churchill Livingstone, 1969)

Close, Sylvia: *The Know-how of Pregnancy and Labour* (Wright, 1975)

— *Birth Report* (National Foundation for Educational Research, 1979)

Dick-Read, Grantley: *Childbirth without Fear* (Piper, 1969)

Karmel, Marjorie: *Babies without Tears* (Secker & Warburg, 1971)

Kitzinger, Sheila: *Birth at Home* (Oxford University Press, 1979)

— *The Experience of Childbirth* (2nd ed: Gollancz, 1972)

— *Giving Birth: Parents' Emotions in Childbirth* (Gollancz/ Sphere, 1971)

Leboyer, Frederick: *Birth without Violence* (Wildwood House/ Fontana, 1975)

Llewellyn-Jones, Derek: *Everywoman: A Gynaecological Guide for Life* (2nd ed: Faber, 1978)

Lux Flanagan, Geraldine: *The First Nine Months of Life* (Heinemann Medical, 1963)

Madders, Jane: *Stress and Relaxation* (Martin, 1979)

Macfarlane, Aidan: *The Psychology of Childbirth* (Fontana/Open Books, 1977)

Milinaire, Caterine: *Birth* (Omnibus, 1976)

Montgomery, Eileen: *At Your Best for Birth and Later* (Wright, 1969)

Nilsson, Lennart et al: *The Everyday Miracle* (Faber/Penguin, 1977)

Wright, Erna: *The New Childbirth* (Tandem, 1969)

POSTNATAL and FEEDING

Close, Sylvia: *The Know-how of Breast-Feeding* (Wright, 1972)

— *The Know-how of Infant Care* (Wright, 1972)

— *The Know-how of Infant Feeding* (Wright, 1973)

Eiger, Marvin S., & Olds, Sally W.: *The Complete Book of Breast-Feeding* (Bantam, 1974)

La Leche League International: *The Womanly Art of Breast-Feeding* (Souvenir Press/Tandem, 1970)

Leboyer, Frederick: *Loving Hands* (Collins, 1977)

Raphael, Dana: *The Tender Gift: Breast-Feeding* (Schocken, 1976)

Stanway, Penny & Andrew: *Breast is Best* (Pan, 1978)

Index